Own Yo

Own Your Cancer

A Take-Charge Guide for the
Recently Diagnosed and Those Who Love Them

Peter Edelstein, MD, FACS, FASCRS

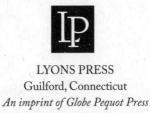

LYONS PRESS
Guilford, Connecticut
An imprint of Globe Pequot Press

Lyons Press is an imprint of Globe Pequot Press.

Text design and layout: Sue Murray
Project editor: Ellen Urban

Library of Congress Cataloging-in-Publication Data

Edelstein, Peter S.
  Own your cancer : a take-charge guide for the recently diagnosed and those who love them / Peter Edelstein, MD, FACS, FASCRS.
    pages cm
  ISBN 978-0-7627-9637-3
  1. Cancer—Popular works. 2. Cancer—Patients—Decision making. I. Title.
  RC263.E33 2014
  616.99'4—dc23

                                                   2013050243

Printed in the United States of America
10 9 8 7 6 5 4 3 2 1

Thanks, Helen.
Thor

Contents

1

Why Did I Buy This Book?

I hate books that begin with definitions. But since I'm not reading this book, tough luck for you (not the worst tough luck you've had recently, I would bet).

"Definitive." It means conclusive, ultimate, from a recognized expert authority. Don't believe me? Look it up online (that's what I did). I had never heard the word "definitive" prior to entering medical school (if I did, it went unregistered, as I was watching football or dreaming of getting to second base with my college girlfriend). Since then, I've heard "definitive" a thousand times. In the pathology lab, in the operating room, in the oncology clinic. Half of the times I've heard "definitive," it has come from my own mouth. "Definitive" is to medicine as "milk" is to Cap'n Crunch cereal. They go together. Especially for physicians whose passion is caring for people with cancer. Given all of the unknowns, challenges, and labile emotions that are part and parcel of caring for people with cancer and their families, we physicians desperately seek the comfort of things that are definitive. We relish X-rays that are definitive in clearly demonstrating "no evidence of cancer spread to the lungs." We're grateful for the definitive pathology report that states in no uncertain terms, "prostate cancer cells are clearly identified." And we especially like to take definitive action. No "Gee, I'm really not sure if you should receive any chemotherapy" for us. Definitive. "I am quite certain that it is clearly appropriate for you to undergo chemotherapy treatment." Definitive is confident. Definitive is sure. Definitive is safe. As cancer docs, we love definitive.

So now you know what "definitive" means and the important role "definitive" plays in oncology (cancer medicine).

Now for the bad news: This book is not meant to give you definitive medical advice. Sorry. I can't give you definitive medical advice. No, not because my publisher's lawyer is standing right behind me vigorously shaking her head (although she is). I can't give you definitive medical advice because I don't know you. Just like I can't tell you where to go for a great meal in Philadelphia. I don't know you (or Philadelphia, for that matter). I don't know if you like Chinese food. I don't know what type of cancer you have or your cancer "stage." I don't know how old you are. I have no idea how much you smoke. I don't have a clue if you have high blood pressure, low blood sugar, or a tendency toward blood clots. Each of you is different from everyone else, both in medical terms (your vital signs, laboratory values, X-rays) and as human beings (husbands and wives, children and parents, hard workers and slackers). Dishing out definitive medical advice requires that I know you as a person with cancer and as a person period. And there's not enough space in my living room for all of you, so don't expect definitive. Got it?

That said, I've spent long hours, often stretching into days and nights without interruption, caring for people with cancer. When you spend that much time hanging out with a specific group of people, you hear things, you see things, you pick up things. Themes, really. Themes shared among a group of unique individuals who are experiencing a common set of challenges. You're privy to emotional conversations between your patients and their spouses. You exchange an understanding look just before your patients drift off into an anesthesia-induced sleep, just before you head out to the operating room sink to scrub for surgery. You literally feel the stress in the room as your patients and their children struggle to make small talk, impeded by unspoken words and fears. Common themes shared by unique individuals as they, and now you, attempt to navigate their way through the unfamiliar, life-altering, life-threatening world of cancer.

Okay, enough. This isn't a Robert Frost poem. The point is this: There is now knowledge that must be mastered, issues that must be raised and dissected, and decisions that must be made, all of which can critically impact your new life as a person with cancer. Knowledge and issues and decisions that are not intuitive. That you may not appreciate or understand without some (or even a great deal of) guidance. Many of you who are newly diagnosed with cancer don't even recognize what these key action items are, let alone understand how to approach them. That's not your fault. Hey, I can remove your large intestine without a hitch, but I have no clue how to change the brake pads on my Toyota, which is also pretty damn important. Thus, many newly diagnosed cancer patients seem to enter into a trance, simply floating right past all of the critical knowledge and issues and decisions that will ultimately determine both their quality of life and their survival, slipping down the stream without a moment's pause, led without question or hesitation by doctors and nurses and technicians and the system. Don't get me wrong, I can see why this happens. Your life just drove into a brick wall, or, to use my previous analogy, your life is headed full-speed into a brick wall and you need new brake pads, and you (like me) have no clue how to replace your old, worn ones. Every single aspect of your life changed in an instant, with three little words: "You have cancer."

To describe how you must feel as "overwhelming" is akin to describing the Grand Canyon as "kinda wide." Overwhelming for you, above all. But also damn overwhelming for your spouse. Your family. Your friends. Cancer. The C Word. That was one big shitload to get hit with. So you're already in a daze, and everyone's feeling incredible pressure to get going with your treatment, but neither you nor your wife or husband nor your family nor your friends knows what the hell that means . . . and there are guides aplenty on this tour. Doctors, nurses, therapists, technicians. The system is actually set up to push you down the assembly line without you making a peep or raising your hand, to drive your care with definitive medical advice. Hell, your input really isn't needed. They say you should get radiation therapy . . . get radiation therapy! They don't suggest that you speak with your wife about your potentially dying, so don't speak with your wife about it! They say you're "Stage III." What does it matter if you don't know what that means, as long as they do! (I know . . . if I laid my sarcasm on any thicker, you'd be wiping it off the page. I've never been accused of being subtle.)

Don't do it. Don't be a passive participant in this, a critical part of your life's journey. I get that you're overwhelmed, and what I'm suggesting in this book may seem like adding even more stress onto you. But suck it up. It's important. It's important that you understand what it means that you're Stage III. It's important that you not only appreciate why they are recommending radiation treatment, but that you agree with that recommendation. It's important to understand why and how to speak with your spouse about the possibility and implications of your dying. All of this and so much

Don't be a passive participant in this, a critical part of your life's journey.

more is important if you are to maintain some semblance of control over your life, of your independence, and of your involvement in the knowledge, the issues, and the decisions that will define both the journey and the outcome of your battle with your cancer.

So, overwhelmed as you are, you need to take a deep breath, roll up your sleeves, and get to work. You need to learn about several medical topics, such as what cancer is, how to pick your doctors, how and why you are "staged," what roles the different treatment modalities (techniques) play, and so on. This book will provide you with a rapid, high-level education on these critical medical topics in a language you'll understand while still appreciating your intelligence. But we'll also discuss nonmedical issues that are just as crucial for you to appreciate and ponder if you are to remain in charge of your life in spite of your disease. Your fear of dying. Who should take out the garbage. Whether you can have sex while undergoing treatment. If you should read about your cancer on the Internet. What your diagnosis means to your family's health. These represent the "human themes" common to all of you who have recently learned that you are harboring a malignancy inside of you.

I've learned a helluva lot from my cancer patients, from their families and friends, and from my physician and nurse colleagues. And I've served countless times as a guide, partner, and friend to my patients, their families, and their friends, bearing witness to their struggles and triumphs as they battle to outwit and outlive their disease and to remain true to themselves during the fight, win or lose. They have been my teachers, and it is their lessons that fill many of the following pages.

This book, therefore, is not meant to give you "definitive medical advice." I did not write this for you as an individual cancer patient. Rather, allow this book to serve as a guide to understanding concepts, issues to be raised, decisions to be made, challenges to address, and "ownership" as they all relate to your cancer.

2

What the Hell Do You Mean, "Own Your Cancer"?

I'm going to assume, given that you've already read up to this first sentence of the second chapter of this book, that either you or someone you love dearly has been diagnosed with cancer. Not impressed with my intelligence yet, huh? Wait, I get better.

Cancer. It's a damn frightening word . . . possibly the most frightening word when directed specifically at you by a guy in a white coat in an overly cool room with a skeleton hanging in the corner. First of all, I am truly sorry that you have cancer. I mean it. True, I don't know you, at least not personally, but I do know you in general. I've had the privilege of caring for hundreds of cancer patients over my career as a surgeon and educator, and while I may not be a clinical genius (ask my wife, who is a brilliant doctor) or life guru (again, ask my wife, and this time she'll be backed up by my daughters), my cancer patients were insightful, honest teachers (whether or not this was their intention), and I am a terrific student. So believe me, even though I've never been diagnosed with cancer myself—as someone whose mother had cancer, whose father had cancer, who has delivered the news to hundreds of men and women and gone on to hold their hands, who has spent countless hours in the operating room doing my damnedest to cure them, as someone who has cried with families when we realized that we had achieved a cure, and as someone who has cried with families when we realized that we had failed to achieve a cure—when I say that I know this damn disease. Cancer is horrible and it's unfair and it's terrifying on every level. Now, with all that said and agreed upon, and now that you've heard the horrible, unfair, terrifying news that you have cancer, there's one thing above all else that you must immediately begin to do regardless of your type and stage of cancer: ***You must own your cancer.***

This strong statement likely raises a number of questions for you:

Is there any tangible proof that this guy actually graduated from an accredited medical school?

Given that she agreed to marry him, is his wife really that "brilliant"?

If I gently wipe off the cover, will they let me return this book?

Please, bear with me.

I know you have cancer, but that's not the same thing as *owning* your cancer. Simply possessing something allows you to take a more passive role than does owning something. Oh, I see . . . some of you who have cancer already have accepted that you have cancer. Sorry . . . same problem. The difference between owning and accepting is much more than semantic. Acceptance is still passive.

That is, I accept that I pay too much in taxes. As a result, I don't really do anything about the situation (other than bitching and moaning and paying). On the other hand, owning is active. I own my home; thus, I am responsible for all that happens in my home, both good and bad, and I have to constantly make decisions to keep my home functioning and livable. I want carpeting in the bathroom? Done. I want a sixty-one-inch plasma-screen TV in the bathroom? Good. The water heater in the hallway closet starts leaking? I replace it. The garage door opener fails? I repair it. A patch of lawn is turning brown? I put in additional sprinkler heads. That's ownership. Get it? It's the same for your cancer. If you do not demand and seize active involvement, if you allow yourself to fall into a passive role through fear or unwillingness to learn, then you will lose control not only of the decisions regarding the treatment of your disease, but of many nonmedical aspects of your life, including (and arguably, most important) the thousands of daily minor decisions and routine activities that, until your diagnosis, you took for granted and that cumulatively make up the substance of your life. That is passive. That is surrender. That is allowing cancer to kill you without a fight. That is not ownership.

> *If you do not demand and seize active involvement, if you allow yourself to fall into a passive role through fear or unwillingness to learn, then you will lose control not only of the decisions regarding the treatment of your disease, but of many nonmedical aspects of your life.*

Let's "get into the weeds," as they say in the South. There are two reasons why owning your cancer is so important: The first relates to treatment decisions and the second impacts your quality of life.

Reason #1: Driving Your Cancer Treatment

Unlike accepting that you have cancer, owning your cancer begins with an understanding of a subtle yet critical reality: that you did not "get" cancer, but that *you made your cancer*. That your cancer is a bunch of your cells made by your body. This may seem a bit obvious, but there's a difference between superficially saying it and honestly believing it. Why is this important? Because if you're walking along the road and a car hits you, breaking both your legs, then you got hit (passive). Even though you suffered the injury, the car's driver is the owner of the horrible event, the responsible party. Someone else did something bad to you. That's how most cancer patients view their disease. Deep down, they know that there is no "driver" to blame, yet they still envision the cancer as alien or foreign in its origin, as if they've been hit by a car driven by cancer, as though the horrible event is owned by someone, anyone, other than themselves. No doubt such a disconnect allows many people to psychologically build a wall around themselves in an effort to deal with the terrible news, but such a perspective can also be paralyzing. It is a passive approach, and taking the victim role leads to impotence in facing the enemy within. Own the fact that your own body screwed up and made these dysfunctional cells that are now growing unchecked inside of you and are threatening your quality of life and, for some of you, your life itself. No one to blame. No one has conscious control over their cellular DNA. So someone has to step up to the plate and deal with things. The owner. *You.*

Ownership means accepting full responsibility for the way things are and, more important, for your future and the future of your cancer. If instead you create a disconnect, a wall between you and your malignancy (the driver), you'll slide into the role of a passive victim. Now, grabbing the victim cloak is not only the easiest path to travel, it may represent an entirely appropriate way to go. After all, with a few notable exceptions, the overwhelming majority of cancer patients did nothing to cause their cancer. They developed cancer seemingly as a result of bad luck and/or crappy genes. Even smokers who get lung cancer after years of sucking down carcinogenic fumes rightfully point out the unfairness of it all, that they have ten friends who are also lifelong smokers who never developed cancer, so where's the equity in that? See? Playing the victim is pretty easy and not altogether unreasonable. But for the cancer patient, for you, arguments of ease and reasonableness must be thrown aside, as allowing your cancer to make you its victim is not the right approach to your goal of making your cancer *your* victim (destroying it, banishing it, making it disappear forever).

Those who choose to be cancer's victims sit and wallow in their own self-pity, focused on the unfairness of it all and, often, on their impending doom. Again, I'm not saying that such feelings are not valid—because they are. They're just not productive. Standing in the middle of a burning room and saying, "I didn't light this fire" and "I'll never make it out" will not increase your chances of being home to share dinner with your family. What I call "actionability" is the reason to own your cancer and shun the victim role. Victims are just that . . . victims. But those who own their cancer are empowered. Empowered to make choices, select actions (and, as important, inactions) in dealing with their cancer in the manner they believe best for themselves and their loved ones. Ownership means acceptance of responsibility and empowerment to drive the process as you see fit, just as you accept responsibility and play an active role in most important things in your life (both positive and negative), such as raising your children or finding a job or caring for an elderly parent. Those who choose to own their cancer, just as those who choose to accept the responsibility of raising their children, are the people in this world who are "whole" and who have the greatest chance of achieving their goals, or at worst, going down swinging.

Ownership means acceptance of responsibility and empowerment to drive the process as you see fit, just as you accept responsibility and play an active role in most important things in your life.

Don't misunderstand . . . as we'll talk about later, owning your cancer, accepting responsibility for decisions regarding your disease, does not necessarily mean choosing any and all treatment options. No. Owning your cancer means seeking knowledge and information, asking and re-asking questions, initiating the hard talks, pushing back against experienced advice, and *leading* your cancer journey according to your views on your life.

Reason #2: Fighting for Your Life

The second reason to own your cancer is more thematic, impacting your quality of life as a whole, not just your medical activities. Simply said, I have seen what happens to my cancer patients who fail to own their cancer: They allow their cancer to own them. If you allow your cancer to own you, you will lose much, much more than a seat at the table when treatment decisions are being made. You will struggle throughout the duration of your treatment (and often afterward) to find pleasure in many of the relationships and activities that were the fabric of your life just days before learning of your diagnosis. You will be obsessed, ruled, owned by this disease. It's not that you will dwell constantly on your cancer and your fears, as that may well be the case even if you choose to own your cancer, particularly before and during the early days of your treatment. It's really a mind-set—an attitude, a perspective. I appreciate that harboring a potentially life-threatening disease within your body sucks in every way imaginable, and that the fears associated with death are overwhelming. But the reason the fear of dying from your cancer is so damn overwhelming and terrifying is that there are so many things in your life that you love and don't wish to give up. By failing to own your cancer you voluntarily lose the things that give your life meaning, abandoning the very thing that you fear ultimately losing: your wonderful life. Do you love watching your children play at the park? Don't you dare let your cancer steal that experience from you (or them).

If anything, my patients who chose to own their cancer have told me that their disease has made them love and appreciate their lives even more. This has been true even for my cancer-owning patients who ultimately died from their malignancies. Don't forget: At its core, your fear is that your cancer will take you away from a life filled with people you love, things you love to do, and dreams you still wish to fulfill. Thus, *it is insane for you to let the fear of losing a life you love result in you voluntarily giving up the life you love*, to lose it all not because you die from your cancer, but simply because you have cancer. Hell, even before you were diagnosed, you knew that someday you were going to die and leave behind your wonderful life. So did you stay home in bed, surrounded by soft pillows, because venturing outside might result in your getting pancaked by a runaway bus? Such is lunatic circular logic. Having cancer cannot be permitted to result in the same loss of a cherished life as dying of cancer would.

Having cancer cannot be permitted to result in the same loss of a cherished life as dying of cancer would.

Voluntarily giving up what only death should steal from you is arguably worse than at least doing all you can, even if it's not enough, to hold on to what you love. Don't do it. *Own your cancer,* don't let your cancer own you. It's your choice.

Listen. I get it. Your cancer is the first thing you think about when you wake up. It's the last thing you think about when (or if) you fall asleep. And between waking and sleeping, you think about it all the time. At least for now. But own that damn cancer!

It is part of your life, but not all of your life. As much as you can, continue to own your life. Go and watch your son's baseball game. Take in a movie with your friend. Grab burgers and fries with your family (having cancer is a great excuse for eating heart-unhealthy foods . . . you can blow off the salads without getting grief). Get in a fight with your ridiculously liberal (or conservative) mother-in-law. I'm not saying it will be wonderful. Hell, you may miss your child's home run because you're thinking about your tumor. You may "wake up" in the middle of the movie without a clue as to why everyone is laughing, because you've been wondering if that pain in your shoulder could be a sign that your disease has spread. You may order a cheeseburger when you hate cheeseburgers because all you're thinking about is your damn cancer. That's all fine. But if you choose to own your cancer, if you commit to trying to keep doing the things you've loved to do your entire life prior to hearing the "C Word," then you will begin to rediscover pleasure in your life, even if initially such wonderful moments are few and far between. And as I said previously, many of my patients' experiences suggest that you may value those "little pleasures" even more than ever before.

All right . . . enough lecturing about owning your cancer. (Trust me, you'll hear more about it throughout this book.) Let's talk about Sentinel Events.

Sentinel Events
Throughout your life, you'll experience a handful of particularly impactful and truly life-altering processes. Your marriage. The birth of your children. Graduating from college. A major job

promotion. Serving in the military. These rare experiences, the way stations on your life's journey, are what I call Sentinel Events, or perhaps more appropriately, Sentinel Journeys, as they rarely if ever are short-term in nature. They may begin suddenly, even unexpectedly, but some take months or years to unravel. All ultimately play significant roles in shaping who you are and who you will become for the duration of your life. At a minimum, Sentinel Events modify your outlook and perspective; more frequently, they alter your life's entire trajectory.

As I often remind my cancer patients early in our relationship, not all Sentinel Events are good. Divorce. Getting fired. The loss of a loved one. These challenging and sometimes tragic life-altering experiences deserve as much attention, respect, and appreciation for their impact on you and your life as do the wonderful Sentinel Events. You got it—being handed a diagnosis of cancer is a big damn Sentinel Event, with a capital "S" and a capital "E." But no matter the outcome, no matter whether you die within a year or forty-three years from now, from the moment you heard "You have cancer," your life's journey was irrevocably and permanently altered. Whether its impact has any silver lining (some cancer patients develop a new appreciation for life that, in retrospect, makes their remaining time on earth, whether brief or long, even sweeter) or whether everything relating to your malignant Sentinel Event is 100 percent bloody awful is not my point here. My point is simpler: We must own our Sentinel Events. Whether good or bad, we must understand, analyze, respect, and appreciate the moment: the birth of your child, divorcing the person you once could not imagine living without, achieving that long-sought goal, losing a meaningful job. And being diagnosed with cancer.

We must own our Sentinel Events. It's easy and fun to own the good ones. And truth be told, it's a no-brainer to own many of those bad ones that somehow threaten us. The best example of the latter is divorce, a Sentinel Event experienced by more than half of you reading this book. When you were getting divorced (or if you have never experienced divorce, think of when a friend or family member was going through it), did you simply give your soon-to-be-ex everything you had? The house? The money? The children? No. You stayed awake nights thinking about it, what led up to this failure, your role in it, your spouse's role in it, how to approach it in the short term, its impact over the long haul, what your friends and family thought, how much it might cost you, the impact on your kids. Even if your divorce took place years ago and no kids were involved and you "parted amicably," your divorce has impacted (not necessarily negatively) your approach to the opposite sex, to commitment, to your finances, to your life. We learn from our bad Sentinel Events through owning them. We dwell on our negative Sentinel Events. We dig into them, we analyze their implications, we act on them, we own them. Get it? Say it with me: *I own my cancer.*

One final thing before we get less esoteric, and if you don't yet suspect that I'm a callous bastard, this may just seal the deal. Remember, this is not diabetes. This is not high blood pressure. This is not emphysema. Those are chronic conditions that impact you directly, regularly, daily over years and even decades. While there may be short periods during which a chronic disease worsens (diabetics may need hospitalization to care for infec-tions, for example), such illnesses have long, progressive courses over the years. Not so of cancer. With a handful of exceptions, such as unaggressive prostate tumors in some patients, unchecked cancers grow and grow and grow and spread and spread . . . and kill you. In a relatively short time (relative to chronic diseases, such as the ones I just mentioned). Thus, even if you have a "slow-growing tumor," you have no time to waste on denial or any other of the Kübler-Ross stages of grief right now, okay? You can deny, you can be pissed off, you can negotiate . . . but later, and in small doses. Not now. Now you've got work to do. Actually, you do need one Kübler-Ross grief stage. The last one: acceptance. But as I've told you repeatedly, you've got to move right through that stage now. Because accepting that you have cancer is not enough. It's just step one. Now it's time for the big move: You have to own your cancer.

3

I've Got Cancer ... What Now?

For pretty much everyone who learns they have cancer, one of the initial emotions that washes over them is helplessness. Sure, within minutes of returning from the doctor's office some of you type-A personalities were shooting off e-mail queries to your cousin the podiatrist or googling "thyroid cancer." But many of you simply slumped into your chair, overwhelmed, helpless. Regardless of your reaction, the same handful of guidelines apply. While obviously lack of action and a failure to educate yourself are the antithesis of owning your cancer, immersing yourself in Internet "facts" and hearsay regarding treatment is arguably as valueless and perhaps even destructively misleading. Remember, the Internet has given us definitive proof of aliens on earth, Bigfoot, and the existence of an Elvis–Hillary Clinton love child. (We'll talk more about the Internet soon.)

So, for you who are sitting in your shower, lost and unable to find any next step to take, listen up. Those other folks, the type-A cancer patients, have at least seized the day and begun to practice cancer ownership. Now it's time for all of you to roll up your sleeves. There is a process, and it's your responsibility to drive that process, because it's your cancer. *The foundation of cancer ownership is education.* But education is a hazardous process, as your new knowledge is only as good as the facts and sources on which it is based.

Let's start by delving into the relationship between the Internet and "facts." The beauty of the Internet is that anyone anywhere can write anything. The horror of the Internet is that anyone anywhere can write anything. Nowhere is this freedom simultaneously more empowering and more dangerous than where the World Wide Web discusses medicine. Patients, hospitals, insurers, whack-jobs, physicians, foreign correspondents, alternative medicine therapists, and hundreds and hundreds of uncredentialed, untrained, and ungodly people are granted the credibility that comes with the written word. Many of my patients jumped onto the Internet before we had a chance to talk about the cancer ownership process, and in doing so, many of these suddenly Internet-educated patients had all their hope sucked out of them. You'd think that every new cancer patient would *find* unrealistic hope in those electronic pages—reports of guaranteed cures, personal sagas of survival, lifesaving "statistics," and the like. But in most cases, the opposite occurs. It is human nature to immediately click on "prognosis" or "survival rates" and, voila, it seems that you're a dead man (or woman) walking. Even though you're possibly (or even likely) not. Or you'll read about the toxic side effects of chemotherapy and swear off any such treatment, even if death is the alternative and even if the chemo discussed would never be offered to you. Jumping to the Internet is fraught with risk based on the likelihood that you'll fail to recognize that you don't know what the hell you're reading about, that you lack all or much of the knowledge required to appropriately filter and interpret all of this general information in order to appropriately apply it to your specific situation. Holy cow—if you looked up "alcohol" on the Internet, you'd swear off drinking forever after reading a website about alcoholism or some guy in a van who got drunk and murdered hookers. *Reading cancer information from unqualified authors is a dangerous activity.* Even reading credible Internet material on survival rates that are specific to stage, cellular grade, DNA activity, hormone sensitivity, you the patient, without having a basic understanding of these concepts will experience a violent, visceral response, as your eyes will affix on the horrific five-year survival of some patients whose type of cancer may be the only thing that they have in common with you. Thus, *reading cancer information from qualified authors when you are not qualified to interpret that information is also a dangerous activity.* It's like me reading on the Internet that a family of four died tragically when their Toyota rolled over on the interstate and then running out and selling my Toyota and forbidding my wife to drive on the interstate. If I simply understood that the driver had fallen asleep at the wheel, I might better appreciate how this relates to me (don't drive when sleepy).

> *Reading cancer information from unqualified authors is a dangerous activity.*

So, should you bail on the Internet and rely solely on your physicians to educate you? No. No way. The Internet can be an amazing, empowering tool for you. Just think about the two Ws: *where* and *when. Where* you find information regarding your cancer is critical and not particularly challenging. Learning about your cancer on the "My Sister Survived Her Liver Cancer by Eating Beans" website is like having your teeth cleaned by a guy who knows a guy who's married to a dental hygienist. Sorry—just dumb. Learn about your cancer by visiting Internet sites created and maintained by internationally recognized cancer institutions, such as those by Memorial Sloan-Kettering Cancer Center (arguably the world's leading cancer center, mskcc.org); MD Anderson Cancer Center (arguably the world's other leading cancer center, mdanderson.org); City of Hope Cancer Center (cityofhope.org); Dana-Farber Cancer Institute (dana-farber.org); Moffitt Cancer Center (moffitt.org); Mayo Clinic Cancer Center (mayoclinic.org); Massachusetts General Hospital (massgeneral.org); Johns Hopkins (hopkinsmedicine.org); Duke Cancer Institute (dukecancerinstitute.org); Cleveland Clinic (my.clevelandclinic.org); Stanford Cancer Institute (cancer.stanford.edu); or that great source of credible information, the American Cancer Society (cancer.org). Get it? Get your Internet information from someone with some damn credibility. From an institution that "writes the books" on cancer. From a *cancer center*.

Now on to the "when." Knowing when to use the Internet as your educational source requires that you truly know and are honest with yourself. If you are the type of person who, once on that credible website, cannot read only the pages for which you are prepared, if you will move on to pages for which you're not yet educated enough to correctly interpret, then don't go to any website until you've learned what you need to first learn: your type of cancer; then (most important) your stage of cancer; and (if available) your cancer cell grade. Additional information and understanding will further benefit some of you, depending on cancer type (for example, hormone receptor status for those of you with breast cancer and Gleason Score for those of you with prostate cancer). I know—what the hell is he talking about? Fear not, cancer owner. Now that you're dedicated to educating yourself, by the end of this book, you will understand cancer stage, cell grade, and many other important terms, and you'll know how to utilize this knowledge.

All that said, here's what I suggest: If the only thing you know right now is that you have cancer, and if you have the personality that will limit your Internet exploration at this time to that general topic (a general description of your type of cancer), go to a credible website and read only the page or pages that provide an overview of your cancer. Learn about how it grows and from what cells it has developed. How common it is (the "prevalence")? Who gets it? How does it present—meaning what are the common complaints that lead to its discovery? Just learn the basics. But don't you dare move on to treatment, recurrence, prognosis, survival . . . not until you are ready, by which I mean, not until you know enough about your specific cancer, your specific stage, and (if available) your cancer cell grade to correctly interpret and incorporate what you are reading. The bottom line: If you have not yet completed your cancer staging evaluation or do not know your cancer stage, do not read any more than that general information website page or you'll likely scare the shit out of yourself and your loved ones, probably needlessly. Just because I know how to drive does not mean it is wise for me to rent a car on my visit to Beijing and drive throughout the Chinese metropolis . . . after all, I don't read Chinese, and I don't even know which side of the road they drive on. Don't know your stage yet? Then don't rent a car in Beijing. Wait for a week or two . . . you'll know your stage long before I can identify the Chinese signs for "merging traffic."

So that's the general 4-1-1 on getting started with your cancer ownership and education. The next chapters are more meaty. Some of them (like the very next one) present nonmedical lessons learned from my patients. Others are straight out of cancer courses taught to medical students and residents, filtered for "what matters" and translated into terms (hopefully) from which intelligent, nonmedical people like you will learn what you need to learn.

4

Keep Wiping Your Own Ass

If there's only one chapter in this entire book that your spouse, parents, best friend, and (older) kids should read, it's this one. Oh, yeah . . . you should read it first.

While cancer patient after cancer patient after cancer patient often expressed the same shared frustration with me, none stated it better than a sixty-something year old man suffering from colon cancer:

> *"For sixty years I've taken care of myself, my brothers and sisters, eventually my parents, and then my own wife and children. A couple of weeks ago you told me I had cancer, and now everybody suddenly thinks I can't wipe my own ass."*

This complaint is repeated by patients suffering from every type of cancer. It's as if immediately upon hearing the "C Word," you become an infant. This process, which I refer to in discussions with cancer patients and their families as infantilization, is driven by love, but really screws things up. As I remind my patients' family and friends, the day before they learned the diagnosis, their loved one wasn't a patient, let alone a cancer patient. He or she was a person, a wife or husband, a mother or father, a daughter or son, a friend. A person who took out the garbage, filled the car with gas, made the kids' lunches, mowed the lawn, and yes, wiped his or her own ass. He or she still played with the grandchildren, watched a ball game, swung the golf clubs, enjoyed a dinner out, and had sex (the luckier ones). All of these activities, even the tedious ones that don't directly provide pleasure, are part of our lives, of who we are. We own them, because we own our lives.

Now, I know that your wife or husband, your kids and your friends all love you. But they've been watching too much TV. On television, all serious illness is the same: Within seconds (or by the time the commercial break is over), the cancer victim can barely get out of bed, struggles to walk, and coughs at the slightest provocation. The television cancer patient fades quickly, right before our eyes (after all, it's only a thirty-minute show . . . twenty-one minutes without ads). The truth is that for the majority of you, this TV scenario is not applicable and never will be. Unlike a heart attack or heart failure, which can rapidly sap your strength and may take weeks to months to recover from, newly diagnosed cancer rarely suddenly drains your life force away. Unlike pneumonia, newly diagnosed cancer rarely triggers horrible, prolonged coughing spells. Unlike kidney failure, newly diagnosed cancer rarely results in the accumulation of fluid that swells the legs and feet and impedes your walking. Thus, unlike your counterpart on TV, you'll notice no monstrous difference in your physical status or capabilities thirty minutes after learning you are a cancer patient than you possessed thirty minutes before learning you are a cancer patient (twenty-one, without commercials).

The explanation for this (other than the time pressure felt by television writers) is that the majority of you who were recently diagnosed do not have cancer that has spread widely throughout your body (what is termed as "disseminated"). That is, your lungs and your liver are not filled with cancer growths (called distant metastases, as discussed in the following chapters). Some of you didn't even know you had cancer until it was seen on a mammogram, felt on a prostate exam, or visualized on a colonoscopy. Given that, why shouldn't you still take out the garbage, let alone enjoy a dinner out? Perform every function the day, week, and month after you learn you have cancer that you performed the day, week, and month before you learned you have cancer. This is how to own your cancer and by doing so, how you *continue to own your life*, as you have for decades.

Perform every function the day, week, and month after you learn you have cancer that you performed the day, week, and month before you learned you have cancer.

Now at the time of your recent cancer diagnosis, some of you may well have had symptoms, such as pain or difficulty breathing. And others of you may develop physical problems that make performing some or all of your pre-cancer routines difficult or impossible. That's okay, and for those activities that are too tiring or truly impossible for you, ask a loved one or a friend for assistance. They'll gladly help you, you'll truly appreciate it, and that's how it's supposed to work. However, this may not be as simple as it sounds. Many of you are used to being "the strong one." The mom. The dad. Tough old Grandpa. You've never needed help, doggone it. *You've* been the helper. To you folks I can only say, it's okay. Asking your son to help you lift a box won't diminish you in his eyes one bit. He loves you, and you love him. Let him help you now, because you need it, just like you helped him when he was a little kid, when he needed it.

Here's the risky part, the slippery slope . . . *don't allow the let-us-help-you floodgates to burst open and infantilize you.* Just because you need (and ask) for help mowing the lawn doesn't mean you can't dress yourself. Sure, get any and all the help you need. But don't allow friends and family to do for you what you can still do yourself. Keep living your life.

Your family and friends won't understand. They're trying to help you, and like you, they're scared about your cancer, scared about what comes next, and then what comes after that. Will you need an operation? Will you need radiation? Will you need chemotherapy? Will you be able to go back to work? Does our insurance cover all this? Will you die? The many, many questions that you have, each potential answer opening the door to another flock of questions, are the same questions filling the minds of those who love you. Later in this book, we'll discuss these questions and how both you and your loved ones can begin to address them. But for now, let's remain focused on preventing your infantilization at the hands of those loved ones who are trying to help you.

Some of my patients tell me visit after visit how angry they are that their family and friends are treating them like infants. Many of these patients feel bad, having even yelled at a loved one who was "just trying to help." It's a fact that well-intentioned people with nothing but love in their hearts can in actuality be taking away yet another part of the daily routine that defines a cancer patient as an independent person still living his or her life. After listening to these tales of anger and frustration, I'd look my patients in the eye and ask, "Why the hell are you telling *me* this?" As they returned a confused look, struggling to understand my rejection, I'd continue. "You should be telling *them*. *They're* the ones who need to know how you feel. They want to help, they're trying to help, and they have no idea that in trying to help, they're not helping." I'm sure that for some of my patients this contorted explanation did little to clear the confusion. But with further discussion, the point was made.

There are two primary explanations as to why your friends and family are infantilizing you, both based on their love for you, but both of which backfire. First of all, when someone you love has cancer, you're frightened both for them and for yourself. Frightened big-time. Such big-time fright is worsened by the feeling of impotence. Everyone's heard the story of the mother who sees her baby trapped under a car tire (I never understand how this happens, but let's continue). She's so overwhelmed by her instinct to save her child that superhuman quantities of adrenaline course through her body, bestowing upon her the strength of a thousand mothers, and she lifts the car off her baby. When those who love you were told that you have cancer, they were like that mother seeing her baby trapped under the tire of a car—but different. Because any moron (let alone any mother) would instinctively know that the baby will be saved only by lifting the car. The lifesaving solution is simple, obvious, and instinctive. Human beings do better addressing big-time fear when we know what the hell to do. Tiger in the kitchen? I'll close the door to the living room and slide the antique cabinet in front. Movie theater on fire? I'll grab the kids and bolt out the side exit. Wife diagnosed with breast cancer? I'll . . . Total and complete impotence. When someone we love has just been told that he or she has cancer, we have no clue "what to do." You have a car tire on your legs, but you're in Texas, and your loved ones are seeing it all on TV from Norway—they feel totally helpless. Which scares them even further.

By taking over your activities, your family and friends are "doing something" to deal with this terrifying situation that threatens you. In fact, they're really doing the only thing they can do (unless they happen to be cancer surgeons or oncologists). They'll do the shopping, take care of the car, pick up the kids, clean the house. They'll get you every meal, prop you up on pillows, bring you the TV remote. Wipe your ass. Thus, the first driver of your infantilization is fear for you, producing this great itch to do something in an effort to scratch and relieve this fear.

The second reason for infantilization is the natural follow-up to the first reason. Not only does doing something make your loved ones feel less impotent and, as a result, slightly less scared (or, perhaps, just distracted from their fear), *they also believe that they are truly helping you.* As I said a few paragraphs ago, diseases like cancer, heart failure, pneumonia . . . these are all lumped together in the minds of most people. You've got a bad disease, so you must be weak, fatigued, unstable. They want to help you.

So, infantilization is the result of two well-meaning processes, the consequence of which for you is anger, frustration, and the loss of ownership of your life. But there is an answer. One solution that simultaneously addresses both causes of the problem. And if you can perform this task, achieve this solution, you've truly demonstrated some cancer ownership. The solution: *Talk openly, honestly, appreciatively, and lovingly to them about what's going on and what you're feeling.* By first thanking them but then explaining why what they're doing for you is actually making you unhappy, the infantilization process will stop dead in its tracks. You'll have destroyed the "wanting to help" cause of the problem by gently informing them that they are not helping. And then by pointing the way for them to truly help you by talking openly and honestly about your and their feelings and fears concerning your cancer, you'll not only benefit, you'll also be providing them with an activity, something they can "do" to feel less impotent. And a bonus: You'll be helping them, too, as you always did before hearing your diagnosis. Now what infant can say that?

So do it. Tell them the truth, that they're infantilizing you. Thank them for the loving intentions behind their actions, but make it end. Assure them that you will ask for help whenever you need it (and do so . . . don't be macho). And then talk with them, telling them that in always being able to talk honestly, they are offering you so much more than their washing the dishes when it's your night at the sink.

As mentioned earlier in the chapter, how and what to discuss with family and friends is a big and important issue for you and for them and something we'll address later in this book.

5

Now the Medical Stuff:
The "Lingo" of Cancer

I've always been bothered when hearing of professional colleagues who explain medical issues (diseases, treatment options,
complications, prognoses) in a way that not only prevents their
patients from understanding what the hell is going on, but also
prevents their patients from participating in their own cancer
care decisions. Hell, I don't let the car salesman determine which
model, what color interior, and my monthly payments when I
buy a new car. So why should you allow your cancer doctors to
exclude you (even unintentionally) from the critical knowledge
and decision-making processes? After all, it's my new car, and it's
your new cancer.

Now don't get me wrong. The majority of my colleagues have
terrific bedside manner and communication skills, especially
those physicians, nurses, and additional clinical providers who
have chosen to specifically care for cancer patients. Those physicians who fail in these efforts do so, I believe, for two primary
reasons, which are not mutually exclusive:

1. Most forget that they are speaking in a "foreign language," that even medical terms that physicians think everyone knows and understands are, in fact, poorly if at all understood (let alone clearly comprehended by a person dealing with a new cancer diagnosis).

2. They assume that their patients are not intelligent enough (which is very different from "not educated enough") to understand the complexity of their current medical situation.

In writing for you here, I'm going to make the same two assumptions I do when speaking to a newly diagnosed cancer patient and his or her family:

1. I assume that you're at least as smart if not smarter than I am.

2. Notwithstanding my first assumption, I am going to assume that you did not go to medical school and then spend years studying cancer.

Based on my two simple yet staggering assumptions, I whole-heartedly believe that after providing you with a couple of important educational cancer lessons, as well as with a short glossary of common cancer terminology, you'll jump to the top of the class and take a major step forward as a cancer owner. We'll start at the beginning.

What the Hell Is Cancer?

A little biology background to start my answer.

Your body is composed of cells. Trillions of cells come together to make up your organs (liver, lung, brain, heart, kidney, pancreas), your skin, your glands (including your mammary glands, or breasts), your bones and ligaments, the whole shebang. Other cells, such as the red and white blood cells racing through your circulation, work solo, functioning individually. All of your cells are programmed to automatically perform their specific duties, whether as part of an organ or structure or as independent contractors, allowing you to live, grow, digest, breathe, sleep, fight infections, have sex, whatever. And throughout your body, many of your cells are programmed to die at genetically triggered times in their (and your) life. Thus, millions of your cells are constantly, and appropriately, dying on a regular basis, committing a sort of cellular suicide in a process known as cellular **apoptosis.** The cells lining your intestinal tract from the inside of your mouth through your rectum turn over rapidly, dying after only a few days of functional life and sloughing off into your stool (yes, every bowel movement is thus like a mass cellular funeral . . . get over it). Blood cells are intentionally removed and destroyed by your body every 120 or so days. Thus many normal, healthy cells have programmed life spans and targeted times for cellular death. Not cancer cells. Cancer cells have lost their programming for cell death. That is, cancer cells are *immortal.*

Another key thing that your cells are programmed to do is to know when to replicate (divide and increase in number) and when to grow or, as important, when to *not* replicate and *not* grow. Finally, your cells know *not to grow into each other.* Here's what I mean by that last statement: You can tightly duct tape your hands together for the next month, but when someone finally removes the sticky binding, your hands will not have grown together. The skin of your left hand will not have grown *into* the skin of your right hand. I promise. (As a side benefit, you'll likely have lost weight, being unable to open a potato chip bag or hold a chili-bacon cheeseburger.) Why don't your hands grow together? After all, when you *cut* your hand, the skin grows back together as you heal. When damaged (as when you cut your skin), cells do rapidly divide and grow, bridging the gap and repairing the wound, until the cells on both sides of the cut grow to contact one another. At that point, when healthy cells are touching (and the wound is closed), those cells stop advancing across the now-nonexistent gap, as normal, healthy cells do not invade (let alone destroy) other cells with which they come into contact. This control over excessive cell growth demonstrated by your skin and other nor-mal cells is called **contact inhibition.**

Let's "paint a picture," shall we? You have a barn that houses twenty farm animals. Your barn holds two horses in a stall, four cows in a paddock, four sheep in a pen, five rabbits in a hutch, and four hens plus a rooster in a coop. In our body-barn analogy, each species of animal has a different function (obviously, the cows are your breasts, and let's have the hens be your liver, horses your kid-neys, or whatever bizarre representations ring your chimes). The barn is big enough to hold all twenty beasts, each species housed within its own enclosure. You're the farmer here. As usual, the rab-bits start multiplying. But unlike in the past, when you removed and sold the baby rabbits, you're vacationing in the Bahamas. The rabbits breed and breed and breed, and soon there's not enough room in their little rabbit hutch, which neighbors the horse stall on one side and sits next to the cow paddock on the other. Unfortunately, you've extended your tropical vacation, so the mass of rabbits continues to grow unabated. Soon, the horde of multiplying, growing, fluffy beasts is so great that they burst through one side of their hutch. The rabbit herd now spreads out a little, and as the young ones grow and new ones are rapidly born, the bunny population spreads and spreads and spreads, pushing against the horse stall on one side of their broken pen and against the cow paddock on the other.

Now wait. You think you got it, don't you? The rabbits are cancer cells, right? Wrong! If it was that easy, medical school would only last three weeks, and you'd allow your farmer to perform your prostate exam.

Cells that grow uncontrollably (the rabbits) may not be cancerous. We all experience uncontrolled cell growth that is **benign** (not cancerous). Common examples of benign growths include fibroids of the uterus (uncontrolled, noncancerous growths of uterine muscle cells) and lipomas (uncontrolled, noncancerous growths of fat cells). Benign growths are called **benign tumors;** cancerous growths are called **malignant tumors.** The overwhelming majority of benign tumors won't kill you; most won't even harm you, and quite a few are only detected unexpectedly on an X-ray or during a physical examination or at autopsy (these are called **incidental findings**). Uterine fibroids, for example, often cause no symptoms at all and are routinely discovered by a gynecologist performing a physical examination or an ultrasound study. However, some uterine fibroids do cause uterine bleeding, produce pain, and/or prevent successful pregnancy, problems requiring medical or surgical treatment. (Surgical removal, whether of a benign tumor or a malignant tumor, is called surgical **resection.**) Lipomas are often discovered as lumps under the skin of the neck or back during routine physical examination. However, on occasion, a lipoma can cause pain (especially if rubbed on by clothing) or create a cosmetic problem. If a benign tumor of the stomach or intestines grows large enough, it can block (obstruct) the intestines or press on important adjacent structures, impeding urine flow, causing nerve pain, or producing other symptoms. In these examples, a benign tumor (noncancerous growth) can be uncomfortable and/or dangerous, requiring treatment.

Much less commonly but much more dramatically, benign brain tumors, even small ones, can cause blindness, seizures, and even death. As our rabbit hutch surrounds and holds in our rabbits (before they multiply and grow out of control), our skulls surround and hold in our brains. But while the rabbit hutch breaks open as the number of rabbits grows, the solid skull does not "give," not even a little, when a benign brain tumor grows. And there's so little extra space within the skull in the first place that even limited tumor growth dramatically increases the pressure within the skull (called **intracranial pressure**). And increased intracranial pressure means increased pressure on the brain itself, causing real problems, such as seizures, blindness, and/or paralysis. If the pressure continues to build, as it inevitably does with the continuing growth of the benign tumor, the brain has nowhere to go other than the small hole at the base of the skull through which the spinal cord passes from the brain down the neck and back. If any of the brain is pushed out this hole, a horrible event called "herniation," the patient dies. From a *benign* tumor.

Okay, let's step back again. Cells that grow uncontrollably, failing to limit their growth or to die as they are programmed to do, are not necessarily cancerous (malignant). They may be benign. So what's different about a benign tumor versus a malignant one? To answer this critical question, we must go back to the farm where up until now the growing mass of rabbits that busted out of its hutch is pressing against the horse stall and cow paddock, acting like a benign tumor. So what would our floppy-eared bunnies act like if they were a malignant (cancerous) tumor? Mean rabbits. I mean really mean rabbits. The malignant rabbits don't just push against the horse stall. They break through the stall's wood railings, rush into the horse stall, and eat the horses. They push into the neighboring cow paddock and do the same. But that's not all—some of the carnivorous, mad rabbits look around and, rather than head to the neighboring horse stall or cow paddock, hop at a frenetic pace across to the other side of the barn, where they begin munching on the hens and the rooster.

While any farmers have likely stopped reading this by now (and are either weeping openly or racing to their barn to eyeball their rabbits), the rest of you need clarification on two key points that differentiate our benign rabbits from our malignant rabbits:

As they grow, malignant cells don't just push against their neighboring normal cells. *Malignant cells have lost their contact inhibition.* Malignant tumors are **invasive,** penetrating into adjacent healthy tissues, and **destructive,** destroying the invaded tissues.

A second distinction: Benign cells don't "travel." When there were too many rabbits to remain within their hutch, the rabbits pushed against the neighboring horse stall and cow paddock. But the malignant rabbits *hopped across the open barn* to attack the hens and rooster. Malignant cells can travel from their origin to non-neighboring structures and then invade, destroy, and grow within their new home. A growth of such traveling cancer cells is called a tumor **metastasis** (a "**met**" in the common vernacular). More than one metastasis are called tumor **metastases** (or "**mets**"). Benign tumors may grow to enormous size (I have on more than one occasion removed a benign tumor the size of a softball from a patient's pelvis), but even gigantic benign tumors remain in the location in which they formed; *benign tumors do not metastasize.* Thus, patients have only one benign tumor, whereas cancer patients have not only the original growth (the **primary tumor,** or "**primary**") but may also harbor one or more mets. Sadly, during many operations, I have found cancerous tumors no larger than my fingernail that have already spread (metastasized), producing dozens and dozens of small and large mets throughout my patient's liver.

And don't forget what you learned previously. While one morning you, the farmer, will stroll into your barn and find your oldest bunny cold and stiff in the hutch, cancer "rabbits" never die. They are immortal creatures that eat other animals . . . very disturbing (unless you're a Hollywood executive).

It is these few unique and powerfully horrible capabilities that make cancer cells the monsters they truly are: the lack of contact inhibition allowing malignant cells to invade and destroy nearby healthy tissues; the potential to travel even great distances within the body, spreading into new tissues through invasion, destruction, and metastatic growth; and, oh yeah, they friggin' live forever.

We'll discuss metastatic cancer spread in greater detail, as well as cancer **recurrence** (reappearance) and other important issues, later in this book.

Cancer has its own language, but whereas you can count on the Italians to speak English during your visit to Venice, you can't count on all your doctors, nurses, therapists, technicians, and other cancer care providers to translate cancer lingo

Understanding the language of cancer is foundational to cancer ownership.

into a language you'll understand. What follows is a simple glossary of additional terms from the world of cancer that we have not yet defined or discussed. Understanding the language of cancer is foundational to cancer ownership. Critical in creating this foundation is your commitment to asking questions. No physician thinks, "What an idiot," and no nurse rolls her eyes, when you ask what a word or phrase means, even if you ask the same question a second time. In reality, such questions and requests for clarification will most likely lead your care providers to apologize, as we are not communicating as clearly as we wish. In fact, it is not uncommon after such clarification requests for a physician's communication skills to dramatically improve. Remember, *there are no dumb questions*, including simply asking for word definitions or general explanations. And if you do feel that the clinician (doctor, nurse, whomever) is judgmental or hostile when you ask a question, you should find a different clinician. You are the one with the cancer.

The Lingo

The following basic terms are commonly used by professionals in the cancer world. Many of these terms are important for you to learn and understand in order to participate in (and drive) your care. Refer to this glossary as frequently as necessary. Many of these terms are discussed in much greater detail elsewhere in this book.

Oncology

The medical term for the field of cancer.

Oncologist

An expert with training specifically in the care and treatment of cancer patients. Oncologists are not surgeons; rather, they have completed training in internal medicine and then completed additional training in oncology. They are the "keepers of the chemotherapy." They recommend specific chemotherapeutic treatments (called **regimens**) for your consideration, administering that chemotherapy to you, monitoring you for side effects, complications, and evidence of successful destruction of your cancer, and following you for years after treatment, diligently searching for the return of any cancer that survived (cancer **recurrence**). For most of you, your oncologist will be the physician with whom you are most engaged during treatment and with whom you will have a long-term relationship.

Growth / Tumor

These terms are often used interchangeably and refer to a group of cells displaying uncontrolled growth. Thus a growth/tumor may be benign or malignant (if the latter, it is further identified as either the primary tumor/growth or a metastatic tumor/growth). A tumor, particularly one of significant size, is also commonly referred to as a **mass** or **lesion**, although the latter term can refer to any abnormality, including non-growth abnormalities such as a gunshot wound, burn, or laceration.

Biopsy

A biopsy can refer to (1) a piece of tissue from a suspected tumor, retrieved to provide the doctor who specializes in this (called a **pathologist**) with a sample to evaluate for evidence of benign or malignant cells or (2) the procedure of taking the tissue sample itself. If a biopsy reveals malignant cells, the pathologist can often also gain additional information, such as the potential aggressiveness of the malignant cells (**cell grade**). Growths that are suspicious for representing primary tumors are biopsied, as are many growths that are suspicious for representing metastases. Today most biopsies are non-surgical, performed by an interventional radiologist or surgeon using a small needle that is passed through your (numbed) skin and into the suspicious growth, often under the guidance of a CAT scan or ultrasound image of that particular area of your body. The needle is used to retrieve a small piece of the suspicious tissue (**percutaneous needle biopsy**). Some biopsies are still performed surgically through an incision when a needle biopsy is not possible or has repeatedly failed to provide a

pathological diagnosis to determine whether cancer is present. Surgical biopsy is also performed if it's determined that complete removal of a small growth will not only provide the pathologist with adequate tissue to diagnose cancer but also represents the total surgical treatment if a cancer is diagnosed (this is called an **excisional biopsy**).

Cell Grade

At its core, cell grade is a determination of the **differentiation** of your cancer cells relative to normal cells of the same type. *Cell grade (differentiation) is an important indicator of the aggressiveness of your cancer in terms of growth and of potential for metastatic spread.* Cell grade is usually categorized numerically, using the numbers 1 through 4, with higher numbers indicating less cellular differentiation and a more aggressive cancer cell profile— meaner rabbits, in our previous farm analogy. Thus for a cell grade, lower numbers are better. The determination of cell grade is made by a pathologist, who examines your cancer cells (sampled via a biopsy or surgical procedure) under the microscope. In addition, many cancer cells are further evaluated by chemical tests (called **immunohistochemical assays**) that evaluate your cancer cells for the presence or absence of certain proteins, and even by analysis of your cancer cell genetic profile (DNA or RNA). No need to get further into these complex diagnostic processes and tests here. Just appreciate that there are often multiple analyses performed on your cancer cells to determine how differentiated they are relative to normal cells of the same tissue, and that this information guides treatment recommendations and **prognosis** (chance of survival). Thus, colon cancer cells harvested by biopsy are compared to normal colon cells, malignant pancreatic cells to normal pancreatic cells, and so on. The less the cancer cells resemble normal cells of the same tissue type, the less differentiated they are, and the higher the cancer cell grade and aggressiveness. Thus "**well differentiated**" cancers are given a lower grade and are seen as less aggressive (less dangerous) than "**moderately well differentiated**" cancers, which in turn are lower grade and less aggressive than "**poorly differentiated**" or "**undifferentiated**" (also called "**anaplastic**") malignancies. These latter grades are the most serious.

Let's use a simple example. If your contractor builds you a house with the foundation poured into the ground, the floors placed where they're supposed to be, the staircases built in the right spots, the kitchen sink in the kitchen, the toilets in the bathrooms, and a solid roof over the whole thing, but the pool is built in the *front* yard instead of where you said to place it in the back yard, that's a "well-differentiated" house. It looks pretty damn close to a normal house, other than the pool being in the wrong yard. If, on the other hand, your contractor goes on a drinking binge and *then* builds your house, the roof may be in the basement, the stairs may go nowhere, the toilets may be in the front yard, and the chimney may be built out of pieces of your swimming pool, all covered by a concrete foundation. It barely resembles a house. That is a "poorly differentiated" house. It is far better to live in a well-differentiated house than in a poorly differentiated house. The same is true for cancers. Well-differentiated (low-grade) cancers are less aggressive in terms of growth and likelihood of metastasis (spread) than are poorly differentiated (high-grade) cancers.

Cancer Stage and Staging

For more details, read the upcoming chapter on this critical issue. For now, understand that your "stage" is an evaluation of all of the specific locations (sites) within your body that harbor cancer, including the primary tumor site and all cancer metastases. Understand that this stage determination represents our best educated guess based on the limits of our medical (and, particularly, radiologic imaging) capabilities. "Staging" is the general process through which you are staged. As you will learn in a subsequent chapter, you will likely receive a **clinical stage** and a **pathological stage.**

Local Versus Regional Versus Distant Disease

We'll really dig into these concepts in an upcoming chapter, but suffice it to say that these three terms are geographical. "Local" represents the site of your primary tumor. "Regional" refers to the physical area and anatomic structures that lie within the area immediately surrounding your primary tumor, most importantly the lymphatic vessels and lymph nodes. "Distant" tends to refer to the remainder of the body other than the local and regional tissues (although as you'll learn in the detailed chapter on staging, there is some crossover).

Hematogenous Spread

Metastatic cancer spread via the bloodstream (circulatory system, vascular system). This is discussed in more detail in an upcoming chapter.

Lymphatic Spread

Metastatic cancer spread via the lymphatic system. Again, this is discussed in more detail in an upcoming chapter.

Resection

This term simply means surgical removal. When a tumor is surgically removed, physicians say the tumor has been "resected."

Margin

Also called the **margin of resection,** the margin is the outside boundary of what is taken out in surgery—the surgical specimen of tumor surrounded by an encasement of normal tissue. (The goal of surgery for a malignant tumor is to remove the cancer within a three-dimensional surrounding layer of normal tissue, which will be discussed in detail in a later chapter.) The pathologist uses a microscope to study very thin slices of the surgically removed tissue to determine whether the removed cancer is entirely surrounded by a rim of healthy tissue, as is the goal of the operation. If all of the cancer is surrounded by an appropriately thick, solid layer of normal tissue, the likelihood that any cancer remains at the site of surgical removal (usually the primary tumor site, but sometimes the site of metastasis cancer spread) is low. For different types of cancers, the thickness of normal surrounding tissue that is removed at surgery in an attempt to cure the patient differs. Thus, a favorable pathology report will state that the surgical specimen had "clean margins," meaning that all of the removed cancer was entirely surrounded by an appropriately thick layer of normal tissue. Much more concerning is a pathology report indicating the presence of "microscopic disease" near or "at the margin," as this suggests that microscopic clusters of cancer cells may well remain within the patient. And far and away the worst report is of "gross disease at the margin," a situation usually known to the surgeon at the time of the operation. (A surgeon often knows that some gross cancer is being left behind, usually accepting this outcome because removal of the entire cancer would be too dangerous or disabling to the patient.) The status of the margins has significant implications for treatment and prognosis.

Treatment

"Treatment" is also routinely referred to as "**therapy.**" When the word is used alone, "treatment" generally means any and all treatments used in an attempt *to cure* a patient. This is as opposed to **palliative treatment** or **palliative therapy,** the important goal of which is to reduce symptoms (such as pain or obstruction) in a patient who is deemed incurable. Treatment may involve surgery and/or radiation therapy and/or chemotherapy, depending particularly on tumor type and stage, but also on cell grade and, often, on other factors. You know what surgery is, and for many cancers, surgery plays the main role in attempted curative treatment. Many patients after undergoing an apparent curative surgical resection have no evidence of any remaining cancer. That said, depending on type, stage, grade, and so on, the likelihood of recurrence may be high enough that **adjuvant treatment** is given even though there is no evidence of remaining cancer. Adjuvant treatment is simply any treatment or treatments provided after an initial treatment that leaves you with no evidence of cancer.

So why use adjuvant treatment (which is discussed in the chapter on treatments)? The recommendation is based on studies that demonstrate an unacceptable likelihood that microscopic cancer cells are actually still alive within the patient despite the lack of detection of any remaining cancer. Clear as mud, right? Listen . . . you left your old tennis shoes in the garage for six months, and when you finally need them again, you notice that there are ants crawling all over them. So you brush the ants off with your hand and look at the shoes again. No ants. *At least none that you can see.* Are you simply gonna slip your bare feet into the shoes? *No way.* These are those damn little black biting ants. So now before you place your feet into your shoes, you try an additional technique, just in case some ants are still running around inside the shoe, hidden from your view. You bang the shoes together. That's adjuvant therapy. The initial treatment (with intent to cure) was when you brushed off the visible ants with your hand. After that, you saw no ants, but the risk of ants still being present was too high (painful bites) relative to the hassle of adjuvant treatment (banging your shoes together). Unlike this ant analogy, in which you might witness additional ants falling out of your shoes as you bang them together, whether any cancer cells survived the initial treatment and were subsequently killed by adjuvant treatment is never known. (Unfortunately, the reverse is not true: When cancer recurs even after adjuvant therapy or in the absence of adjuvant therapy, it's clear that cancer cells survived the initial treatment.) Adjuvant therapy may be in the form of chemotherapy and/or radiation therapy. *The determination of whether or not adjuvant therapy is appropriate is not always straightforward.* If there is a big difference in survival between those who do and those who do not receive adjuvant therapy, then adjuvant therapy may be favored. But what is a "big difference"? Is a 92 percent chance of surviving five years after adjuvant treatment a "big difference" compared to an 89 percent chance of surviving five years without adjuvant treatment? And before you answer, factor in that adjuvant treatment is associated with the risk of toxic side effects. Is that 3 percent improvement in five-year survival worth six months of nausea and the risk of life-threatening infections? These numbers and this example of toxicity is just that: an example to make a point. That point is that *you must weigh the benefits versus the risks of adjuvant therapy.* And to make such a crucial judgment, you have to understand all that is involved.

Neoadjuvant therapy is related to, but different than adjuvant therapy in its timing of delivery—before surgery. For example, we learned awhile ago that many rectal cancer patients had an improved chance of cure if they received adjuvant therapy following their surgical cancer resection. That is, even though we could find no remaining rectal cancer after surgery, the addition of chemotherapy and radiation therapy increased their chance of being cured. Then someone got the brilliant idea that those rectal cancer patients should receive some of their adjuvant therapy not after, but *before* their surgery. Why? Why not wait for the surgeon to first remove the big tumor mass and then give the chemotherapy and radiation? It turns out that for this and some other types of cancer, the radiation appears to be more effective in killing cancer cells *before* the surgeon has destroyed the blood vessel network that supplies the cancer cells; that is, radiation may be more damaging to the rectal cancer cells if the cancer's own blood vessel system is still intact. And the simultaneous administration of certain chemotherapy drugs further enhances the killing effect of the radiation. The final bonus is that many rectal cancers are so damaged by this neoadjuvant chemotherapy and radiation that the tumors greatly shrink, allowing the surgeon to more easily remove the cancer, and even allowing some patients to avoid a permanent colostomy (in which the intestine is brought to the skin and drains stool into a bag attached to the abdominal wall). Pretty good stuff, huh?

Chemotherapy

Routinely referred to as "**chemo**," chemotherapy is cancer treatment (for cure or as adjuvant, neoadjuvant, or palliative therapy) using medications (**chemotherapeutic drugs, pharmaceuticals, agents**). Administered **intravenously** (into your vein), **orally** (swallowed), or sometimes via injections or internal pumps, these drugs target cancer cells for destruction. However, their toxicity frequently also affects normal tissues, resulting in toxic side effects and potential complications. Nausea, loss of hair, and fatigue represent side effects that are bothersome (often very bothersome). Infections and other toxic problems are more than bothersome; they can be dangerous complications. That said, there are a number of medications aimed at reducing the impact of side effects, and some chemotherapy has only rare, mild, or even no side effects. It is common for a patient to receive more than one chemotherapeutic drug, and the combination of chemo agents (which may include several drugs at differing times) is called the chemotherapy **regimen.** Oncologists are the physician experts regarding all things chemotherapy. Chemo is discussed in detail in an upcoming chapter.

Radiation Therapy

Referred to simply as "**radiation,**" this treatment uses radiation energy to damage cellular DNA, killing the targeted cells. Because this killing technique is not cancer-specific, normal, healthy cells are often as vulnerable as malignant cells to radiation's destructive force. Thus, radiation equipment and the delivery of **XRT** (the shorthand for radiation therapy) has evolved into an amazing array of treatments aimed at maximizing radiation energy's impact on tumor cells while minimizing injury to surrounding normal tissues. While the many types and approaches to radiation treatment are beyond the scope of this book, its two main forms are external (or **external beam**) and internal (**brachytherapy**) radiation treatment. In the former, equipment outside of the patient delivers the radiation directly through the body, guided by radiologic images and targeting the cancer within. In the latter, radioactive material (in forms such as small pellets or seeds) is temporarily placed within or immediately adjacent to the tumor within the body itself. Radiation may be used as a curative treatment or as palliative, adjuvant, or neoadjuvant treatment. You'll learn more about XRT in an upcoming chapter.

Recurrence

This term is really a **misnomer** (descriptively incorrect) in that cancer "recurrence" sounds as if the cancer was eradicated and then magically reappeared. In reality, cancer recurrence represents the visible identification of one or more cancer growths that *survived treatment* and were initially too small to identify. The "recurrence" frequently represents metastatic groups of cells that survived treatment, were too small to see prior to and/or immediately following treatment, and then continued growing until they were finally identified. For example, all radiographic imaging studies (X-rays, CAT scans, etc.) may fail to identify small clusters of metastatic breast cancer cells growing within the liver or lungs following treatment, and for the next months or even few years, the patient and her physicians may, therefore, believe that she has been cured. Eventually, however, she will be diagnosed with a **metastatic recurrence** of her breast cancer. Recurrence may also result from hidden cancer cells that survive at the site of the original primary tumor. For example, following initial surgical treatment for rectal cancer, a small deposit of viable rectal cancer cells may remain. If recognized by the surgeon and/or pathologist, the patient may receive radiation therapy to the pelvis in an attempt to kill the remaining tumor cells. Whether or not recognized and treated, if some of these cells survive and grow, they will eventually be discovered and diagnosed as a **local recurrence** of the rectal cancer. Recurrences (metastatic and local) are eventually detected when they grow to a size at which the recurrent cancer is seen on an X-ray or CAT scan, or to a size that causes symptoms (such as bone metastases causing bone pain), or to numbers that allow for detection of substances released into the bloodstream by the cancer cells (such as the PSA protein produced by some prostate cancers or the CEA protein associated with some colon cancers).

Prognosis

Prognosis is a scientific understanding of the track record of patients with a specific type and stage of cancer over a defined period of time. *Simply said, your prognosis is your chance of survival.* Thus the prognosis of Stage III rectal cancer patients describes how many patients with Stage III rectal cancer die from their disease, are alive but still have rectal cancer (at the primary site and/or metastatic disease), or are alive and cancer-free at specified years following initial diagnosis. **Five-year survival** is a common prognostic time period, as for many cancers, a patient is deemed cured if they are alive and without any evidence of remaining or recurring cancer five years after first being treated. (For other cancers, "cure" is applied after a shorter or longer period of time has passed, but five-year survival is a common standard.) Given that prognosis is stratified by cancer type and cancer stage (and, for some cancers, also by cancer cell grade and other features), *the only prognosis that has any validity for you is the prognosis for your type of cancer and your stage of cancer (and any other relevant features).* This is very important. In addition, your individual prognosis may be impacted by your overall health. For example, a Stage III low-grade (differentiated) thyroid tumor may have a worse prognosis in an elderly patient with severe heart failure and emphysema, as such a person may have more difficulty tolerating treatment than an otherwise healthy and younger individual. Such specific health and demographic information about you as an individual does not, of course, make its way into books or website prognosis pages. Thus, when you look up or hear your prognosis, remember that such a prognosis does not include health factors specific to you. For that just-for-you-prognosis, you'll need to speak to your physicians—and even they may disagree or simply quote the same literature that you have read.

Simply said, your prognosis is your chance of survival.

Your Cancer

This is not a medical term but rather a generic and dynamic term. When used in discussions with you (delivered by physicians and other clinicians, and even when you are speaking to others about your disease), "your cancer" refers to *your total cancer burden*. That is, if your cancer is confined to your primary tumor, your primary tumor represents *your cancer*. When you have one or more metastases, regardless of what organ or organs the mets are growing within, "your cancer" refers to your primary tumor plus all of your metastases. If after your primary tumor has been removed, you develop one or more mets, "your cancer" now means your total metastases. Once you're believed to have had all of "your cancer" removed and/or treated, when there is no evidence that you have *any* cancer left in your body, you may still receive adjuvant treatment or simply be followed to make certain that you don't experience a recurrence. In this

scenario, the term "your cancer" refers to the total cancer burden that you had *prior to treatment*. Even thirty-two years after
you're cured, you will tell others that "your cancer" is cured.
Think about those two words (no, not "is cured," although those
are wonderful words): your cancer. If those two words don't des-
ignate *ownership*, I don't know what does.

6

I Hope You Haven't Met:
How Cancer Spreads

As you now know, cancer cells can travel, a process known as cancer metastasis. The two primary routes by which malignant cells metastasize is through the vascular (or circulatory) system (the bloodstream) and through the lymphatic system. While metastatic tumors can themselves serve as the source of additional metastatic cells, for the most part when we think of metastatic cancer, we are thinking of metastases whose cells originated in (and traveled from) the primary tumor.

Cancer Spread via the Bloodstream ("Hematogenous Spread")

The cells that make up your malignant tumor are similar to your healthy cells in one critical way: They all depend on an adequate blood supply to survive. As do all cells living within your body, cancer cells need the oxygen and nutrients brought by arteries (blood vessels that carry that bright red blood away from your heart and lungs to the rest of your body) and require carbon dioxide and other byproducts to be carried away by veins (the thin, low pressure blood vessels that carry that dark blue blood back to your heart and lungs). Malignant tumors are incredibly crafty in their selfish drive for immortality, producing and releasing substances that stimulate the rapid growth of new blood vessels to the tumor (a process known as **angiogenesis**), thus supporting their ongoing, uncontrolled growth. As the medical community has begun to decipher the genetic and protein pathways involved in angiogenesis, several new drugs have been developed and commercialized that specifically work to inhibit angiogenesis; that is, they block some part or parts of the chemical pathway that malignant cells use to trick the body into growing new blood vessels to serve the tumor. Thus, not only do malignant tumors depend on blood vessels for survival and growth, many tumors actually drive the production of more and more blood vessel growth to them. A fringe benefit of these numerous tumor blood vessels (from the cancer's perspective) is that they provide the individual cancer cells access to your entire body. It's like living on an entrance ramp to the interstate. Your circulatory (vascular) system is your body's network of highways and surface streets. From any one point in your body, an individual cell can travel to almost any other site by catching a ride in the bloodstream. That said, it is rare for cancer cells to successfully metastasize to and grow within most parts of the body. How can that be? The answer is that the distant spread of cancer is far more complicated than simple access. I'll get into this very important issue after first discussing cancer spread through the lymphatic system.

Cancer Spread via the Lymphatic System

What the hell is a lymphatic system? You probably already know what lymph nodes are—those large, movable lumps under your chin and in your neck that you've felt when you've woken with a horrible sore throat. They hurt when you press on them, rolling painfully under your probing fingers. Or perhaps you've felt similar tender lumps in your armpit after developing an infection in a cut or a cat scratch on your arm or hand. Or in your groin, when you've had an infected scratch or cut on your thigh or lower leg. Lymph nodes are the "train stations" on the railroad network that is the body's lymphatic system. Without delving too deep, the cells of our body are constantly bathed in fluid, appropriately called "extracellular fluid." Extracellular fluid is fluid that is continuously leaking out of the circulating blood within our blood vessels. Cells push water, salts, and molecular substances out into the extracellular fluid as well. If our extracellular fluid was not "drained away," we'd all swell up and explode (well, maybe not explode, but we'd certainly all have to buy XXL clothes). The extracellular fluid drainage control system is the lymphatic system. A complex network of low pressure, low volume lymphatic vessels (much, much smaller and much, much more fragile than blood vessels) is present throughout your body, shadowing your circulatory system. Extracellular fluid enters into these lymphatic vessels (**lymphatics**) through the tiny pores (openings) in the lymphatic vessel walls. Once within the lymphatics, the fluid is called **lymphatic fluid.** Along with the fluid, numerous and varied types of immune cells flow within the lymphatic vessels, gaining critical access to sites of infections and injury. Similar to blood-carrying veins, smaller lymphatic vessels merge into fewer, larger lymphatics, and these merge into even fewer, larger lymphatics. Ultimately, all of the lymphatic fluid enters one of two lymphatic vessels (though they are the largest in the body, both are still quite small), which drain over three liters of lymphatic fluid a day back into the heart. Thus, your body is one big circulating system, just like your swimming pool filtration system. Much of the fluid that leaks out of the bloodstream and is pushed out of your cells into the extracellular fluid is ultimately carried back and returned to the bloodstream via the lymphatics. More than three liters a day . . . try drinking three liters of anything in a day. Pretty damn impressive for tiny, fragile lymphatic vessels, eh?

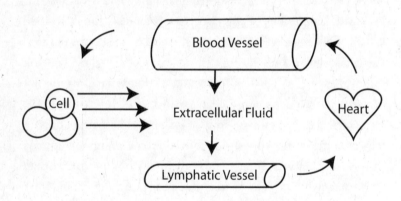

A primary function of our lymphatic system is the identification and destruction of **foreign bodies,** such as bacteria and viruses. That's why when you have an infection (sore throat, infected cut, whatever), your lymphatic system kicks into overdrive and attacks the invading foreign bodies. In this state, your "train stations" (lymph nodes) often swell near the site of the infection, as that is where your body has amassed its army of immune cells to destroy the invading hordes. But this immune function is not limited to bacteria and viruses. Our immune system is programmed to identify damaged and "foreign" cells as well. It is precisely as a result of our immune cells' vigilant search for foreign cells that organ transplant patients must regularly receive strong **immunosuppressant drugs.** Otherwise a transplant recipient's own immune cells would attack the transplanted organ, seeing it as foreign, leading to transplant rejection. But let's get back to cancer. Cancer cells can enter the lymph system through lymphatic vessels surrounding the tumor, just like they can enter the circulatory system. As we'll discuss in the next couple of paragraphs, cancer cells traveling via the lymphatic vessels routinely become trapped in the lymph nodes. There, clever immune cells may see proteins on these cancer cells that are not found on normal cells, thus identifying the cancer cells as foreign. But some cancer cells are able to fool your immune cells, appearing to be your normal cells by hiding the features that would identify them as different and dangerous. (We'll discuss this aspect of **malignant potential** later in this chapter.)

So, we need our lymphatic system, or else we'd likely die as babies the very first time we ate the dog's poop (and certainly during college, when we scarfed down highly questionable pizza on a nightly basis). But despite its vigilance, the lymphatic system is, for many cancer cells, the easiest route for spread. Lymphatic vessels are numerous and surround our tissues. Their walls are **porous** (easily passed through). And the lymphatic fluid within them flows slowly. Thus, entering the lymphatic stream is often the first malignant metastatic spread that occurs. But unlike spread via the bloodstream, *metastatic spread through the lymphatics is frequently somewhat sequential and predictable.* This is because all along the network of merging lymphatic vessels (think railroad tracks) are lymph nodes (like train stations). When a cancer cell enters a lymphatic vessel, it flows with the lymphatic fluid to the first downstream lymph node. Lymph nodes are complex filters within which foreign bodies (bacteria, viruses, cells) are filtered from the fluid and trapped for evaluation by immune cells residing within the lymph nodes, and (if recognized as foreign) attacked and destroyed by the immune cells, a process you notice as painful swelling of the nodes. Cancer cells are routinely filtered out of the lymph fluid at the first lymph node (or one of the first nodes) through which they pass, usually very near the primary tumor. However, one of the most important characteristics of some cancer cells (which we previously touched upon and will again) is their ability to "fool" our immune cells into seeing them as "normal," thus avoiding immune cell attack and destruction. That immune cells within a lymph node don't recognize, let alone attack, many cancer cells explains why physicians are relieved when a patient comes in complaining of a painful lymph node; painful lymph nodes harbor immune cells attacking foreign bodies. Thus, painful, enlarged lymph nodes almost never contain cancer. Painful, enlarged nodes are almost always associated with benign infections. Physicians are worried by *painless* enlarged lymph nodes. Because once trapped within a lymph node but under no attack from immune cells, cancer cells do what they do best . . . they grow, and grow, and grow. Thus, *painless enlarging lymph nodes are worrisome*. And at some point, there are enough cancer cells within the node that one or more of them is able to pass out of the filter system that is the node and continue flowing within the lymphatic fluid, traveling until filtered out by one of the next lymph nodes down the line, where the process repeats itself.

While it is likely that some cancer will metastasize to the liver, lungs, and other organs via lymphatic spread (if the cells make their way back into the bloodstream after the lymphatic fluid drains into the heart), the overwhelming majority of non–lymph node metastases reach their targets via the bloodstream. Lymphatic metastatic spread is usually confined to the lymph nodes, often nodes near but occasionally nodes located far from the primary tumor.

Understanding these basics of lymphatic metastasis will help you understand what we'll discuss in more detail later: your cancer staging (identifying all the locations within your body harboring cancer) and the surgical collection and pathological analysis of your lymph nodes.

Why Doesn't Every Cancer Patient Get Mets?

So, cancer cells are constantly shedding into your bloodstream and traveling throughout your body. And cancer cells are regularly passing into your lymphatic system and moving from lymph node to lymph node. Then *why doesn't every cancer patient develop tumor metastases?* Because while such vascular and/ or lymphatic access is necessary for cancer to travel and grow away from the primary tumor, cancer-specific factors play the primary role in determining the likelihood of successful metastatic spread.

A critical factor in understanding your cancer's likelihood of spreading is your tumor's **metastatic potential.** Metastatic potential means exactly that: the potential of your cancer cells to successfully travel to, invade, and grow within a location apart from the primary tumor site. First of all, *different types of cancers have different malignant potential.* Think of it this way: We both have cars, so we both have the same potential to travel from the South Side of Chicago to O'Hare Airport, right? Wrong. My car is a 1972 AMC Gremlin with only a half-gallon of gas in the tank (and sadly, an eight-track tape player). Your car is a brand-spanking-new Porsche 918 Spyder with a full tank of gas (and a six-disc CD player). Only you will successfully travel from the South Side to O'Hare. I will not (I'm out of gas, with crappy music). Just because we both have cars doesn't mean our cars have the same "potential" to travel. And just because you have bladder cancer does not mean that your bladder cancer has the same metastatic potential as the pancreatic cancer growing inside some other guy. In fact, the difference in metastatic potential between differing tumor types may be significant. Some types of cancers tend to be much more aggressive in metastasizing—these cancers have "greater" metastatic potential. For example, many **sarcomas** (cancers arising from tissues such as muscle, fat, bone, blood vessels, nerves, and the like) are "high grade" (poorly differentiated; aggressive; see the previous chapter on Cancer Lingo). Many of these sarcomas possess big-time metastatic potential and require aggressive treatment *even if no metastases are detected at the time* *of initial treatment*, as microscopic metastases are presumed to be present within the liver or lungs but simply too small to be seen on CAT scan or X-rays. Small cell lung cancer is another malignancy with whopping metastatic potential, often **presenting** (first being diagnosed) with metastases throughout the lung. Thus, understanding the general metastatic potential of your type of cancer (thyroid, liver, lung, breast, whatever) is important in understanding your treatment options and prognosis.

While certain types of cancer routinely have greater metastatic potential than other types, *even two cancers of the same type may display different metastatic potential.* This difference is often reflected in the cell grade, where less cell differentiation (and thus higher grade) is an indica-

> ***Even two cancers of the same type may display different metastatic potential.***

tion of greater metastatic potential. (If you've forgotten about cell grade, return to the Cancer Lingo section at the end of Chapter 5.) The combination of tumor type and cell grade strongly suggests overall metastatic potential and, for some cancers, additional cellular features, including genetic activity, also are used in this determination. This individual cancer cell variability in metastatic potential explains a common source of confusion for my medical students assisting me during surgery: Upon finding an enormous colon cancer, I would often let out a thankful sigh of relief. No, I'm not a sadist. No, I didn't collect my surgical fee prior to the operation. Just the opposite. As I'd explain to my students, for a colon cancer to reach such a size suggests that the malignant cells possess minimal metastatic potential. Why? Because colon cancer cells with greater metastatic potential will likely succeed in spreading long before the primary tumor achieves a large size. So many tumor cells are regularly entering the bloodstream that those with significant metastatic potential may successfully spread to distant organs while the primary tumor is still small. As I said in a previous chapter, I have on several occasions in the operating room found a small primary cancer the size of my fingernail and a liver filled with dozens of mets. Thus, a small tumor may or may not have cells with significant metastatic potential, but finding a very large primary tumor often suggests limited metastatic potential. See? Size really does matter, and sadly, even when talking about primary tumors, bigger is better.

Metastatic potential is cancer cell specific because cancers, even if of the same type, often differ in tumor cell grade and other features that play a role in malignant spread. As discussed previously, your cell grade is determined by pathological examination of a small sample of your cancer cells to determine how similar (low grade and better for you) or dissimilar (higher grade and worse for you) those cells are from normal cells of the same tissue type. (Again, feel free to return to the glossary at the end of Chapter 5.) The less differentiated the cancer cells (classified as a higher number on a range from 1 through 4), the more aggressive the cancer in terms of growth and metastatic potential. Thus, colon cancer cells harvested by biopsy are compared to normal colon cells, malignant pancreatic cells to normal pancreatic cells, and so on. The less the cancer cells resemble normal cells of the same tissue type, the less differentiated they are, and the higher the cancer cell grade and aggressiveness (which translates into more aggressive local growth and greater metastatic potential). Your gastric (stomach) cancer may be well differentiated (which would be good) while your neighbor's gastric cancer may be poorly differentiated (not good for your neighbor).

Again, other cancer-related factors in addition to malignant cell type and grade impact metastatic potential. As noted previously in this chapter, some cancer cells are able to "fool" immune cells within the body—particularly immune cells stationed within lymph nodes—into being seen as normal and, therefore, are allowed to survive without attack. However, we don't have tests that can easily tell us which cancer cells are skilled at fooling immune cells and which are not, even though it's an important component of metastatic potential. As discussed earlier, **angiogenesis** (the ability of cancer cells to initiate new blood vessel growth to support themselves) is also a critical aspect of metastatic potential.

One thing that might be confusing to you is why, in a tumor composed of millions and millions of cells, I am talking about metastatic potential as if it is the same for every one of those cells. Because most scientists believe that *cancers almost always arise from a single cell*. The development of a malignant tumor from a single cell is called **monoclonal carcinogenesis** (from a single cell, the development of cancer). The theory of monoclonal carcinogenesis postulates that *all of the malignant cells within your tumor are clones, identical to one another and to the original cancerous cell*. While there may be some minor differences between cells as a result of additional mistakes that occur during cellular replication (mutations), in general terms it is appropriate to think of all of your millions and millions of cancer cells, whether in the primary tumor or in tumor metastases, as being copies of the original. Therefore, in general, *each of your cancer cells has the same potential for metastatic spread*. This means it is unlikely for a tumor that has little metastatic potential today to develop significant metastatic potential next week or next month.

So now you know why we usually treat a high-grade sarcoma patient more aggressively than a low-grade thyroid patient: Treatment recommendations are based on the differing metastatic potentials of the two tumor types and cell grades. (In our car analogy, both patients have cars, but the sarcoma is a far-traveling, aggressive Porsche and the thyroid cancer is not-fit-to-travel Gremlin . . . the only time in history you'd rather have a Gremlin than a Porsche.) It also explains why we may be less aggressive in treating a patient with a low-grade colon cancer (grade 1 or 2) than a patient with a grade 3 or 4 colon cancer. (In this auto analogy, both patients own Chevrolets, but the first owns a Chevy Malibu and the second owns a Corvette.)

In summary, when trying to understand your cancer's metastatic potential:

- If you had or currently have cancer metastases, you already know your cancer's malignant potential: It's high.

- If you've developed mets after a "curative" treatment, most commonly surgery plus chemo, and with or without radiation (that is, if your cancer has "recurred"), you already know your cancer's malignant potential: It's high.

- If as of today you have never had any known spread of your cancer (regardless of whether your primary tumor has yet been treated), then the first indicator of your cancer's metastatic potential is the *type* of cancer you have, and the second indicator is your *cell grade*.

There are uncommon exceptions to this summation, but they do not merit further discussion here.

While metastatic potential is critical in determining the *likelihood* of your cancer spreading, it is not the sole factor in determining *where* your cancer is likely to spread. If it was, tumors with big-time metastatic potential would grow everywhere (liver, lungs, kidneys, eyes, tongue, thighs, and so on). In reality, certain organs and body structures are much, much more commonly the target of metastatic cancer spread. In addition, specific types of cancer tend to target specific organs and structures for metastatic spread. For the purposes of this discussion, we are talking about hematogenous (bloodstream), not lymphatic, metastatic spread.

The liver and lungs are the most common organs in which mets are found. Enormous volumes of blood flow through the liver and lungs. Both organs have very dense microcirculation (microscopic blood vessel networks), critical to the liver and lungs carrying out their normal functions. In addition to the vast amount of blood that is regularly passing through the liver and lungs, the structure and architecture of these two organs make the liver and lungs, for lack of a better real-world analogy, like your kitchen sponge. While you can hold your sponge under a stream of water flowing from the faucet, the sponge traps that water, and that water moves slowly through the sponge, getting caught up in the little pathways before ultimately dripping out of multiple sites on the other side. Imagine that the water coming out of your faucet contains thousands of microscopic grains of sand within it. Many of those grains would enter the sponge and become trapped, never coming out the other side. While the liver and lungs are different from each other in their density and other features, for those of us who have operated on both, the sand-sponge analogy is a reasonable way for you to think of how malignant cells get trapped in these two organs. Thus, the quantity of circulating tumor cells regularly passing through the liver and lungs is significant relative to most other organs and body structures, and the architecture of these organs may further the likelihood of "trapping" traveling malignant cells.

While the liver and lungs are frequent metastatic sites, specific cancer types also target specific body sites for metastatic spread. The "Seed and Soil" theory suggests that traveling cancer cells are most likely to gain a foothold and survive within a tissue target similar in critical chemical ways to their original primary tumor environment. Whether this theory is correct or not, we know that this cancer type–specific metastatic targeting is real. Thus, in addition to the liver and lungs, breast cancer favors the bones for metastatic spread. Prostate cancer, too, has a propensity for bone metastasis. Stomach cancer is relatively unique in targeting the ovaries for metastatic spread in female patients. And other tumors also have very specific metastatic target profiles.

And then there's renal cell carcinoma, the most common type of kidney cancer. Every medical student learns that "renal cell cancer can metastasize *anywhere*." This is a bit dramatic as, like most cancers, renal cell cancer metastasizes most frequently to the liver, lungs, and bone (and lymph nodes), followed by the brain. However, this unique malignancy has also been reported to, rarely, spread to a wide variety of unusual locations, including the eye, the inside of the nose and the adjacent sinuses, the tongue, the tonsils, to glands (such as the thyroid and parotid gland), the skin, and even to the heart.

Still, for the majority of you, the organs and structures that will be most important to evaluate prior to treatment and to study regularly in follow-up when searching for recurrent cancer are your liver and lungs. Bones are a third site of study for many of you, and your brain is also worth keeping an eye on for a smaller number of you. In addition, *learn whether your cancer tends to target an organ or structure* not on the above list. As the owner of your cancer, you gotta learn and know this stuff.

＊＊＊

Let's summarize the key points regarding cancer metastases that you have learned in this chapter.

- Amazing as it seems (and is), the millions of cells that compose your cancer are all the same as each other, all clones of one original malignant cell. So in general, all of your cancer cells have the same metastatic potential. This means that each of your individual cancer cells possesses (or lacks) the same tools necessary for travel through the bloodstream and/or lymphatics, invasion of distant tissues, "fooling" your immune cells into leaving them alone, and triggering your body into rapidly growing new blood vessels to sustain the growing met.

- In general, different types of cancers have different metastatic potential.

- Cancers of the same type often have differing metastatic potentials, resulting from differing cell grades as well as other factors that are not easily measured, such as the ability to "fool" immune cells and the power of angiogenesis to promote new blood vessel growth.

- Most organs and body structures do not see metastatic growth. The most common organs to foster mets are the liver and lungs. In addition, many cancer types spread to the bones. Fewer metastasize to the brain. And certain specific cancers metastasize to other unique sites. Learn where your specific type of cancer goes.

- And only in the cancer-analogy world would you rather own a '72 Gremlin than a Porsche Spyder.

7

Just Look at a Map:
How Your Cancer Is Staged

Fair warning: This is the most "medical" chapter in this book. As such, it can be fairly intense and challenging to understand. Yet the information in this chapter is vitally important if you are to own your cancer, guide your treatment decisions, and continue to live your life. There's no need to read it all in one sitting (hell, even I took a break for dinner when writing it). Read some, then put it down. Come back later and read some more, then put it down. And there's no rule that says you can read this chapter only once. Some parts may immediately make sense to you. Others may require reading, thinking, and reading again. Don't worry about it. Learn it. Own it.

❧

It may not be intuitive, but oncology is really a helluva lot like real estate. Whether you're planning on owning a new home or owning a new cancer, it's all about location, location, location. There are two general approaches to understanding cancer location, one more general and the other more specific. While the two approaches relate in several ways, they also differ in significant ways, and both will play important roles as you and your doctors determine and plan your treatment.

The Local-Regional-Distant Approach

We'll begin with the more general approach to your cancer's location. At the highest level, when considering treatment options, physicians (and thus you, as the owner of your cancer) speak in terms of "local," "regional," and "distant" disease. In this sense, understanding your cancer is really a geographical issue. Think of this as a way of "mapping" your disease, similar to your viewing a map of the United States. I live in Florida (yep, humidity, mosquitoes the size of small birds, and lots of old people; but on the other hand, great fishing, warm winters, and I'm the young guy). Think of Florida as the definition of "local." Local refers to the anatomic site within your body in which your primary tumor developed (and, if yet to be treated, still resides). The right or left ovary is the local site in which an ovarian cancer develops. The right lower lobe of the lung is the local site in which some lung cancers arise, while others develop in the left upper lobe or other specific sites within one of the lungs. The local site of a breast cancer may be the upper, outer quadrant of the right breast, the lower inner quadrant of the left breast, and so on (we segment the breast into quadrants plus the breast tissue around and underneath the nipple). As you'll appreciate later in this chapter, the evaluation of your local cancer (primary tumor) is critical to staging and treatment planning and differs based largely on your specific tumor type.

Now, Florida, as you well know, is in the southeastern United States. Think of the southeastern United States as the "region" in which I live. An ovarian cancer arising from the right ovary (the local site) also lives in a region: the pelvis. A left lower lobe lung cancer (the local site) lives in the region of left chest (the left "hemi-thorax"). A right upper outer quadrant breast cancer (the local site) lives in a region that includes the entire right breast and the tissues of the adjacent armpit ("axilla"). Thus, the local site of your primary tumor (Florida) is within the region (southeastern United States) of your primary tumor. Along with Florida, the southeastern United States region includes several states, thousands of cities, numerous counties, surface roads, highways, railroad systems, rivers, lakes, and so on and so forth. The same holds true for anatomic (body) regions. For example, the pelvic region (the structures and organs within the pelvis) includes part of the colon and the rectum (segments of the large intestine); the uterus and fallopian tubes and ovaries (in women); the prostate (in men); the bladder; vast numbers of large and small blood vessels, nerves, and muscles; pelvic bones; and numerous other structures. The thorax (the chest) has tens of thousands of blood vessels and bronchioles (breathing tubes); lung tissue; pleura (the lining of the lungs and inner chest wall); nerves; lymphatics; and many other tissues. The breast and axilla (armpit) contain skin; muscles; fat; blood vessels; nerves; glandular tissue;

The evaluation of your local cancer (primary tumor) is critical to staging and treatment planning and differs based largely on your specific tumor type.

and lots more stuff. Thus, like the southeastern United States, the regions of the body, one of which includes the local site in which your cancer developed, are filled with a huge number of varied structures. And common to virtually all regions (the brain and spinal cord being notable exceptions) is a vast, complex network of lymphatic vessels and lymph nodes. As you've already learned, the lymphatic system in general and the lymph nodes in particular are critical in the metastatic cancer spread process. While your cancer may spread directly to any of the neighboring organs and structures within the region containing the primary tumor, *the metastatic status of your regional lymph nodes is far and away the most critical aspect in the evaluation of your regional disease.*

So the local site is in the region, as Florida is in the southeastern United States. Finally, look at the entire United States map. The entire country represents the body, and all of the United States other than the southeastern region represents potential sites for distant metastatic spread. Thus, the local site of an ovarian cancer may be the left ovary, in which case that cancer is within the pelvic region, which may or may not contain metastatic lymph nodes and/or direct tumor spread into other pelvic regional structures. But the spread of that ovarian cancer to the lung or liver represents "distant spread," as these organs are outside of the pelvic region. Likewise, a primary tumor in the upper outer quadrant of the right breast (local disease) may spread regionally to the lymph nodes of the right axilla (armpit) and may also metastasize to the liver, lungs, bone, or other distant site.

This terminology is often a source of great confusion to patients and families. For example, many people say that they have liver cancer when, in fact, they have colon cancer that has metastasized (spread) to the liver. True liver cancer arises from a malignant *liver* cell. And I've often heard that a man has bone cancer when, it reality (and much, much more commonly), he has prostate cancer that has metastasized to the bones. Thus, it is the local site, *the origin of your tumor*, that defines what cancer "you have," regardless of any regional and/or distant spread.

Seems easy, right? Well, at times it can be a little less clear. For example, the "ascending colon" is a portion of the large intestine that travels up the right side within your abdomen. Thus, an ascending colon cancer (the local site of disease) lies within the abdominal region. Included in the abdominal region, in fact neighboring (and even touching) the ascending colon is the liver. In some patients, an ascending colon cancer grows so large that the tumor can grow directly into the liver, which represents *regional disease* through "direct invasion." Much, much more commonly, however, the ascending colon cancer spreads to the neighboring liver through the bloodstream (hematogenous spread), which represents *distant* metastasis. This is an example where an organ (the liver, here) can be the target of regional or distant metastatic spread based not on location, but on the route through which the cancer arrives and invades the targeted organ. So my United States map analogy wasn't exactly perfect when I said that "distant" spread was everywhere in the United States *other than* the

> *It is the local site, the origin of your tumor, that defines what type of cancer "you have," regardless of any regional and/or distant spread.*

southeast region. In some cases, "distant" spread can be present in an organ or structure that is still *within* the region. It's as if Alabama is *not* in the southeastern region of the United States (which would make a number of college football fans in Florida very happy), while at the same time Alabama *is* in the southeastern region. Again, that's because in reality, we consider "regional disease" to be present

1. if there is metastatic disease within one or more regional lymph nodes;

2. less commonly, if the primary tumor has directly grown into (invaded) neighboring ("adjacent") non-lymphatic organs or structures; and/or

3. least commonly and specific to a limited number of tumors, separate little malignant growths (called "satellite lesions") are present on other non-lymphatic tissues within the region.

And we consider "distant disease" to be present when cancer is found

1. in lymph nodes, organs, and/or structures outside the region of the primary tumor; and/or

2. in non-lymphatic organs or structures within the region where the presence of tumor spread is not the result of either direct invasion or satellite lesions (virtually always the result of hematogenous spread).

So if it's a lymph node in Alabama, it's regional. If it's anything else in Alabama (liver, lungs, bone, etc.), it's most likely distant spread.

Trying to Determine Cancer Location

As I said in the opening of this chapter, this first general concept in cancer location, "local-regional-distant," plays a role in determining and planning your treatment. That's because the only way to beat (and often simply control) your cancer is by attacking your disease at every site within your body where it exists—that is, by targeting all of the cancer on your personal local-regional-distant body map. If you treat the local disease (primary tumor) but ignore any regional or distant disease . . . well, you get it. But here's the damn tricky part: The locality of the primary tumor is almost always known (only a small number of patients present with widely metastatic disease but no clear primary tumor site), and surgery is highly successful both in evaluating regional structures and in providing lymph node tissue for assessment of regional disease. However, determining the presence or absence of viable cancer cells at every potential distant metastatic site is extremely challenging.

Initially (as we'll discuss further, below), we use CAT scans, X-rays, and other radiologic imaging studies to search for distant cancer metastases in the most common sites of distant spread (based on your tumor type) and at any site where symptoms have arisen (for example, bone pain) or signs have developed (such as a recent change in blood tests that indicates worsening liver function). But the problem is that small clusters of cancer cells living and growing in the liver, lung, bone, brain, or other distant site may be invisible to our technology, even with the rapid improvement in imaging equipment and techniques. Thus, thousands of cancer cells growing as a "microscopic met" often remain undetected, leading to a falsely optimistic assessment of a patient's cancer. In some patients, no doubt there are dozens of unseen "micro mets" at the time of initial evaluation.

For those of you who, unknown to you or your doctors, harbor micro-metastatic disease, only when one or more mets grow large enough to cause symptoms or be spotted on an imaging study or via a blood test (less commonly) or during a physical examination (least commonly) will you know for certain that you have distant metastatic disease. This is a real bummer, reminiscent of the Salem Witch Trials. To determine whether a woman was a witch, she would (or so the story goes) be tied to a chair that was then dunked in the well. Witches would survive the minutes of submersion, in which case the witch would be burned alive. If you were fortunate enough to prove that you were not a witch . . . well, that meant you had drowned. Neither outcome sounds that rewarding. Same for you. It's not "you have distant cancer spread" or "you don't have distant cancer spread"; it's (unfortunately) that you either *know* you have distant cancer spread (which sucks) or you *don't know* whether you have distant cancer spread (and have to wait, often years, to finally know). That said, if no distant mets are found, it's very possible (and with many tumor types, very likely) that you truly do not harbor any micro-metastatic distant disease . . . a great situation, just one that you can't be sure of for a while. And although both the real witches and the non-witches died during their evaluations, the finding of distant metastases, while a helluva lot more concerning than the absence of distant disease, does not necessarily mean you're going to die from your cancer, at least not today, as distant spread may be controllable, and a small number of people with metastatic disease may still achieve a cure. So perhaps the witch trials aren't the best analogy, but you get the point: You either know for certain that you have distant mets and that beating your cancer will be much more challenging, or you don't know whether you have distant (micro) mets, in which case, as we'll discuss later, you and your physicians will have to make some educated decisions in considering chemotherapy treatment.

Simply remember this: Negative imaging studies, absence of symptoms, normal blood tests, and a normal physical examination do not mean that distant microscopic metastatic disease is not already present within your body. I don't mean to depress you. But you own your cancer, so I'm gonna tell you straight up what you need to know. And I'll say it again for emphasis: Many of you in whom no distant cancer spread has been or will be identified in fact do *not* harbor distant cancer spread and have a great shot at cure! So celebrate a "negative metastatic workup," but do so with a healthy dose of cynicism (unless you are fortunate enough to have one of the several cancer types in which distant micro mets and post-treatment cancer recurrence are extremely rare, in which case ditch most of the cynicism and simply celebrate). Such cynicism is, in fact, the main reason that you will be so closely followed up by your physicians for many years after completing your initial treatment. They (and you) are searching for something they and you hope not to find: gross (non-microscopic) metastatic tumors that survived as micro mets during your initial treatment but which have, with time, finally grown to a detectable size. This is metastatic "recurrence" (again, a poor word, given that it never truly disappeared before recurring), and this is the leading cause of cancer deaths in patients who had no distant disease identified when initially treated.

Staging: The Foundation of Your Cancer Treatment

While local-regional-distant is a general approach used in evaluating your cancer and determining your treatment options, **staging** is the specific approach used in treatment planning and foundational in the understanding of your personal cancer. Thus, developing a rudimentary appreciation of cancer staging is critical for you, the owner of your cancer.

Staging evaluates you as an individual cancer patient and describes *how advanced your cancer is*. Staging is a static "photograph" of all of the cancer within you at a single point in time—that is, your **cancer burden.** Most often staging is performed prior to your receiving any treatment; however, patients may be **re-staged** following treatment. This initial staging "photo" of your cancer will play the key role in guiding your treatment.

Staging evaluates you as an individual cancer patient and describes how advanced your cancer is.

In addition, your stage is the main indicator of your chance of cure.

Here's how the staging approach—which is specific to you and your type of cancer—relates to the more general local-regional-distant approach: Your staging photo analyzes your tumor *locally* (the primary tumor), details any *regional* disease, and evaluates the specifics of any *distant* metastases. Thus the general and the specific approaches to mapping your cancer are related. However, staging is much more detailed and specific and plays a much, much more meaningful role for you as a cancer owner.

As I initially explained, staging determines how advanced your cancer is and is an indicator of your chance of cure. These are the politically correct terms. More bluntly (and by now you know that I'm a bit blunt), your cancer stage determines the likely outcome of your battle; that is, the likelihood that your cancer will recur following treatment or even kill you in the immediate future—in other words, your **prognosis.** From these predictions, you'll appreciate how much you'll have to endure in terms of treatment and treatment-related side effects and complications, how worried you'll need to be about your cancer recurring in the years immediately following treatment, and for a few of you, whether this is a battle you even can win. Listen, you're a big girl or boy, you've already stepped up and owned your cancer, and it's not like the concept of dying from your cancer hasn't already occurred to you, so we're just gonna talk plainly here.

Far and away the most accepted and utilized staging format is called **TNM staging.** TNM staging is based on the evaluation of three features of your cancer: the **local tumor** ("T"); the absence or presence of any **regional lymph node metastasis** ("N"); and the absence or presence of any **distant metastasis** ("M"). Thus, TNM staging is an evaluation of your tumor-nodes-distant mets. Again, you can see the relationship between the local-regional-distant and the TNM staging approaches to understanding all of the cancer within your body. However, it is your rigorously evaluated TNM stage that will drive your doctors' treatment recommendations and your treatment decisions as the cancer owner. For the majority of cancers, Roman numerals 0, I, II, III, and IV are used to categorize progressively more advanced cancer stages. That is, the more advanced your cancer, the greater the stage and the higher the Roman numeral (up to the highest, Stage IV), and the more difficult your challenge will be.

Your overall cancer stage is based upon a combination of your T stage, your N stage, and your M stage. Each of these three components, in turn, has its own stage. *As with your overall stage, a lower T stage, N stage, and M stage number is better.*

It's extremely important that you understand that each type of cancer has its own TNM stag-

Each type of cancer has its own TNM staging system.

ing system. If you have pancreatic cancer, your TNM staging system and the implications of each stage are unique, entirely different, and unrelated to the reader who owns a breast cancer. Thus, there is no meaningful relationship between a Stage II *rectal* cancer and a Stage II *bladder* cancer. Apples and oranges (or rectums and bladders, to be more precise). A Stage III *uterine cancer* has meaning only in regards to the treatment and the prognosis (cure and recurrence rates) of *uterine cancers*. A Stage III uterine cancer is less advanced than a Stage IV uterine cancer and more advanced than a Stage 0, I, or II uterine cancer but cannot be compared in any meaningful way to any stage of any other type of cancer. For example, the five-year survival of treated Stage III anal cancer patients exceeds 40 percent, whereas, sadly, the five-year survival for patients owning Stage III pancreatic cancers is only about 3 percent. Staging and the implications of staging are cancer-type specific, got it? Keep the rectums with the rectums.

Now, some of you will have been staged at the time you were initially diagnosed with cancer. Others of you were (or are being) staged very soon after learning that you owned a cancer. For the majority of cancer types, staging most heavily relies upon **radiologic imaging studies.** "Imaging" includes any one or more of a variety of studies, such as CAT scans, MRI studies, ultrasound imaging, and old-fashioned "plain films" (basic X-rays), all generally, and incorrectly, lumped together by nonmedical folks as "X-rays." Staging also frequently includes collecting multiple tubes of your blood to be analyzed in a search for changes that may suggest the presence of cancer spread to a distant organ or structure. In reality, the value of such initial staging blood work in suggesting distant disease is extremely limited. (Blood tests play a more important role following treatment for certain types of cancer that release unique proteins; in such cases, the finding of elevated levels of proteins in the blood may signal cancer recurrence.) Finally, if not performed when you were initially diagnosed (which it should have been), you will undergo a **biopsy** (harvesting of a small piece of tissue) of the suspicious primary tumor growth to allow a pathologist to definitively confirm the diagnosis of cancer. Even if the initial imaging study leaves no doubt that you have cancer, a biopsy is necessary for two reasons:

1. Even a "sure thing" X-ray is still a *picture* of an abnormality, whereas a piece of the tumor is a piece of the tumor.

2. At least for now, the only way to determine cell grade and other cellular features is via analysis of actual tumor tissue.

I've already said that TNM staging is cancer-type specific. In most cases this is particularly true for the T and the N portions of staging. T (tumor) stage depends on the type of tumor you own. For example, rectal cancer arises from a malignant cell within the inside lining of the rectum (the lining in contact with passing stool), and T stage is based on the depth of cancer invasion into the bowel wall, regardless of overall tumor size. Thus, a very large rectal cancer that has only minimally invaded deeper into the wall of the rectum has a lower T stage (and better prognosis) than a very small rectal cancer that has burrowed through the entire thickness of the bowel wall. The T stage of pancreatic cancer, on the other hand, is partially based on the greatest dimension of the tumor. Thus, a pancreatic tumor that is 2.1cm in its greatest measured dimension is a higher T stage than a similar pancreatic cancer that is 1.9cm (only 0.2cm smaller). How do we know that different types of cancer should be T staged differently? That is, why does size matter in determining prognosis for a pancreatic cancer but not for a rectal cancer? And how do we know how to separate the stages for any one type of cancer? I mean, how do we know where to draw the lines for different stages when measuring various cancers? Again, because tens and hundreds of thousands of patients cared for by thousands of physicians have taught us so much about different cancer-specific features and factors associated with prognosis—that is, we understand much about the potential for different cancers to kill their owners (there I go being blunt again). For rectal cancer, it turns out from all those rectal cancer patients who have gone before that depth of tumor invasion into the bowel wall is critical; for pancreatic cancer, tumor size is critical.

Appreciating that your T stage depends on your cancer type also explains why your T staging may involve different types of imaging studies from those used to stage someone else with another type of cancer. An ultrasound study is the best way to see how deeply into the rectal wall a rectal cancer has invaded. So if you have rectal cancer, you should undergo an ultrasound study using a small probe that is passed through your anus and into your rectum. If you have pancreatic cancer, you'll likely undergo a CAT scan of your abdomen, which is the best way to measure the size of your tumor. Your T staging approach is specific to your type of cancer.

As first touched upon a few paragraphs ago, there are several T stage categories for each type of cancer, and each set of T stages is specific to one type of cancer. Thus, the deeper a rectal cancer invades into the bowel wall, the higher the T stage number and the worse the associated prognosis. Likewise, the larger the pancreatic cancer dimension, the higher the T stage number. Thus, every type of cancer has its own T staging criteria, but for all cancers, the lower your T stage number, the better.

Every type of cancer has its own T staging criteria, but for all cancers, the lower your T stage number, the better.

While different cancers have different N (lymph node) stages, and thus your N staging criteria are also specific to your type of cancer, there is far less variability in N staging than in T staging. Unlike T staging—in which depth of tumor invasion, greatest tumor dimension, or some other tumor-specific characteristics determine T stage—at its core, N staging asks one binary ("yes or no") question: Have malignant cells traveled from your primary tumor to a regional lymph node? Now, determining the absence or presence of living cancer cells within any regional lymph node (that is, finding a lymph node metastasis) is often much more challenging than measuring a tumor's depth of invasion or greatest dimension. As you recall, T stage can usually be determined based on imaging studies (CAT scan, ultrasound, etc.). Figuring out whether malignant cells are residing within any one regional lymph node is not so simple. If one or more nodes do contain cancer cells, they may appear larger than other, normal regional lymph nodes on an imaging study only if those cancer cells have grown to large enough numbers. Such lymph node enlargement is at present the only way to identify metastatic lymph nodes on a CAT scan (most frequently), ultrasound, or other imaging study. However, *even the finding of an enlarged lymph node on an imaging study is not a guarantee that the enlarged lymph node truly represents a cancer metastasis*. Lymph nodes enlarge for numerous reasons, many of which are benign. So while the identification on an imaging study of an enlarged lymph node in the region of a cancer is indeed highly suspicious for a lymph node met, N staging has such a major impact on overall TNM staging (and, therefore, plays such an important role in guiding your treatment options and prognosis) that the suggestion of a lymph node met on only an imaging study may be too questionable for you and your doctors. Thus, an enlarged lymph node in the region of a primary tumor is reported as "highly suspicious for a metastatic lymph node" but is not commonly accepted as definitive evidence of malignant spread to the lymph nodes. Only when an imaging study demonstrates numerous enlarged lymph nodes in a typical metastatic pattern in the region of some types of tumors will the radiologist say definitively that lymph node mets are present.

On the other end of the metastatic spectrum, lymph nodes may harbor thousands of metastatic malignant cells without an increase in size that is noticeable on an imaging study. Thus, *the absence of any enlarged lymph nodes on all imaging studies absolutely, positively does not mean that you have no metastatic spread to your regional lymph nodes.* So while T staging routinely provides a result you can "take to the bank," when no enlarged lymph nodes are found on imaging studies, that doesn't necessarily mean that there is no cancer spread to the lymph nodes.

And as said before, even the finding of enlarged nodes doesn't mean that there is cancer spread. So what do you do if one or more enlarged lymph nodes "suspicious for metastatic cancer" are found on an imaging study during your staging? For many of you, your physician will then recommend a biopsy of the suspicious node. Biopsies, which take a small sample of tissue, are usually performed by numbing your skin with a "pain killer" injection and then passing a needle through the numbed skin and into the suspicious node, guided by imaging studies (if the enlarged node is superficial and can easily be felt just under the skin, such as a node in the groin or neck, no imaging guidance is needed). The "interventional radiologist" who performs the procedure draws tissue from within the enlarged lymph node into the biopsy needle, removes the needle from your body, and delivers the tissue sample to the pathologist, who studies the tissue for evidence of malignant cells. Sometimes there isn't enough tissue in the biopsy for the pathologist to give you an answer, and sometimes the pathologist finds no cancer cells and a second biopsy is performed, particularly if the imaging study was "very suspicious," because the biopsy needle may have missed the cancer growing within the node. A "positive biopsy," meaning that metastatic cancer is identified, is definitive for cancer spread to a regional lymph node. Much less commonly, a small surgery is performed to entirely remove a suspicious lymph node for pathological examination (this rare "surgical excisional biopsy" is usually performed on groin and other very superficial enlarged nodes). Surgical excisional biopsy delivers the entire suspicious lymph node to the pathologist for examination; thus, if no cancer cells are found, you are certain that there is no metastatic disease in that node.

How are you N staged if no enlarged, suspicious lymph nodes are seen on your imaging studies, given that such a result does not mean that you don't have small groups of cancer cells within those "normal" nodes? Or what if your lymph node needle biopsy is negative? You may still have other lymph nodes with cancer that are simply still too small to be seen as "suspicious." Whenever your initial staging evaluation fails to find any evidence of lymph node cancer spread, the final determination of your N stage has to wait until your surgical treatment removes the regional nodes for complete examination by the pathologist. This gets into an important area: your **clinical stage** versus your **pathological stage,** which we'll discuss in greater detail soon. Suffice it to say that if your imaging studies are "negative" for suspicious lymph node disease (or if biopsy of suspicious nodes was "negative" for metastatic disease), the answer to the one binary lymph node staging question is "No," and your N stage is "N0." If your N stage is N0, have a glass of champagne. It is not absolute proof that you don't have lymph node metastases, but it's a damn good start.

If, on the other hand, biopsy of your enlarged, suspicious lymph nodes is "positive" in finding metastatic cancer cells, we routinely say that you are "lymph node positive." *Owning a lymph node positive cancer does not mean you are going to die from your cancer.* (Please re-read that last sentence repeatedly until you truly understand it.) While we call lymph node negative patients N0, we don't routinely call lymph node positive patients "N1" because, as with T staging, there are often numerous lymph node positive stages, each cancer-type specific. (For example, "N1," "N2," and so on based on metastatic features such as the number of metastatic lymph nodes and/or the location of metastatic nodes relative to the primary tumor.) Thus *final N staging must again wait until after surgery*, when the pathologist examines all of the surgically removed lymph nodes.

Now, on to M staging. Your M (distant metastasis) stage is the most critical aspect of staging in terms of your likelihood of surviving your cancer's aggressive growth. As with lymph node staging, determining the M stage begins with the binary question: Do you or don't you have distant metastases? Unlike T or N staging, M stage has only two categories for virtually all cancers: You are either "M0" (no evidence of distant cancer spread) or "M1" (positive distant cancer spread). In other words, the finding of distant metastases does not lead to more detailed stratification of M stage based on number of mets, location of mets, or any other features of your distant disease. Despite this lack of staging stratification, differences in location and number of distant mets have significant implications for treatment recommendations, as some patients with distant cancer spread may today survive—with a meaningful quality of life—for years rather than weeks or months when treated with new chemotherapeutic drugs, and a small set of patients with distant metastatic disease may still be cured of their cancer (with surgical resection of their minimal metastatic disease).

As you may recall, distant spread is best thought of as spread via the bloodstream, as opposed to spread resulting from direct growth of the primary tumor or lymphatic spread to the regional nodes. As detailed in the previous chapter on metastatic spread, far and away the most common targets of distant spread are the liver and the lungs. Another frequent distant target is bone (any bone or bones, but most often the spine, ribs, and pelvic bones). Remember that these and other less common distant targets tend to be cancer-type specific, so you'll need to learn whether your particular type of cancer will try to spread to your brain, ovaries, or other sites. I know this is scary, but the more you "know thy enemy," the better prepared you will be to "defeat thy enemy."

Your M staging will almost always include a CAT scan (or similar study) of your abdomen to evaluate your liver. You will also at least undergo a chest X-ray (and possibly a chest CAT scan) to search your lungs for anything suspicious for metastatic cancer. Furthermore, if indicated based on the type of cancer you own, you may receive a CAT scan or MRI study of your brain, a "bone scan" evaluation of your skeleton, a pelvic CAT scan or ultrasound to look at your ovaries, and so on and so forth. Finally, if you have any specific complaints, such as a relatively focal (confined to one spot or area) pain, a bump or growth, a change in your balance, vision, stride (walk), a cough, blood in your urine or stool, altered vaginal bleeding, anything—*tell your physician* so that an imaging study can be performed to evaluate the problem site for metastatic disease. And it doesn't have to be something new. If six months ago you began noticing that one area on your rib or ribs ached a little at the end of the day, tell your doctor. If four months ago you began to occasionally experience a few moments of blurred vision, tell your doctor. Remember, there's no harm, and there should be no embarrassment, in telling your cancer doctors anything and everything that is concerning you. So what if it turns out to be nothing? No harm, no foul. But if it *is* something, and if you *don't* mention it, you may not be offered the best treatment options for treating your cancer.

The reality is that some people are afraid to mention that new symptom, afraid that it *is* a cancer met. But trust me on this one: Being afraid that the new lump in your groin is a cancer met and not telling your doctor about it is not an effective treatment of the cancer met in your groin. Ignoring it will not make it go away.

If your physician finds something that is potentially concerning when examining you (such as a new small bump under your arm or a bone that is tender when pressed), don't you want that "something" evaluated? Of course you do, and so does your physician, and further studies will be performed to make certain that the finding is not metastatic cancer. If it is, while that sucks, it's critical that it was found so that appropriate treatment can be considered.

Finally, in addition to imaging studies, blood tests are also frequently performed during M staging. As said previously, the utility of blood tests in M staging is minimal. Almost always, by the time metastatic disease has advanced to the point where your liver function impairment or bone damage is significant enough to alter your blood tests, your metastatic disease has already been detected via imaging studies and/or your body will have already told you (through new pain, bleeding, a yellowing of the whites of your eyes, significant weight loss, or in some other manner) that you have metastatic disease. And even in the very rare occasion when a blood test is performed early and is found to be abnormal, this leads to . . . a CAT scan, which was soon going to be performed anyway. Blood tests are still routinely performed, and there are at least two good reasons they should be done at the time of your initial staging. First of all, such initial blood tests provide a "baseline" as to how your body is functioning (your liver and kidneys in particular, but other aspects, such as blood level, are broadly evaluated). A baseline appreciation of your health status is important prior to surgery and/or chemotherapy treatment, just as is a baseline physical examination, which will also be performed. Your doctors will compare "how you're doing" after surgery and throughout your chemotherapy and follow-up period to this baseline evaluation. Significant deviations in your blood tests and/or physical examination will trigger investigative imaging studies to search for infections, recurrent cancer, or some other explanation as to why things have changed. Why do you measure your children on the bathroom wall every birthday? Because humans like to compare things against how they were. So getting a baseline on you through blood tests and physical examination is important.

The second reason to draw blood from you during staging applies to a subset of cancer types. Some cancers produce proteins that are released into the blood and can be detected by special blood tests when elevated high enough (CEA produced by some colon cancers and PSA produced by some prostate cancers are a couple of examples). If you have such a cancer, and if your baseline blood test demonstrates the elevated protein, blood will again be analyzed after your treatment. You hope that soon after treatment (often after surgery alone), the cancer-released protein is no longer found in your blood, suggesting that all of the cancer has been removed. If the blood still has abnormally high levels of the protein, you'll undergo additional imaging studies and possibly further biopsies, as this suggests that you still harbor malignant disease. If your blood protein level drops to normal, suggesting that you've been cured (yippee!), you'll have your blood analyzed regularly for the next several years, as *a return of abnormal elevated blood protein levels may well be the first indication of recurrent cancer*. So you can see, for certain cancers, taking your blood at the time of initial staging (baseline) and then again following treatment and yet again through years of follow-up (the latter referred to as "surveillance") may be very helpful and important. Baseline function and surveillance are the two reasons that it makes sense to let them pull vial after vial of the red liquid from your arm during staging, even though it is highly unlikely that the stolen blood will impact the staging itself.

I said that when staging regional lymph nodes (N staging), imaging studies alone aren't always definitive, and "suspicious" lymph nodes are often biopsied so that a pathologist can examine a tissue sample for evidence of metastatic cancer cells. Similarly, the finding of a growth (a "lesion") on an imaging study that is "suspicious for distant metastatic cancer" may require a biopsy (again, often performed nonsurgically with a needle) to determine whether indeed the growth is a distant metastasis. However, biopsy is used to confirm distant metastatic disease much less frequently than to confirm lymph node metastasis. Why? Because, remember, many things other than cancer can lead to lymph node enlargement. Furthermore, the difference in size between an enlarged lymph node and a normal lymph node can be relatively small and somewhat subjective. But the finding on a CAT scan of multiple, solid growths within your liver or lungs or brain, or the identification on a chest X-ray of a growth destroying your rib, is enough to definitively call the presence of distant metastatic disease. So for many distant mets, imaging studies alone are definitive, and no additional tests are required to correctly state that this represents M1 stage disease. As with N staging, if biopsy is required to further evaluate a suspicious distant lesion, the finding of cancer in the biopsy specimen confirms M1 stage, whereas *the absence of cancer in a biopsy of a suspicious lesion does not necessarily mean M0 stage,* as the biopsy may have failed to capture malignant tissue and will likely need to be repeated.

Putting T, N, and M Together: Staging Your Cancer

So you'll have your tumor staged (T), your regional lymph nodes staged (N), and the rest of you staged for distant disease (M). Your individual T, N, and M stages are combined into one global TNM stage that defines your prognosis and your treatment options. The process can be very complex, given that the staging of many cancer types includes multiple substages for T and N (and rarely M) staging. Not only are the T and N components of staging routinely further divided into multiple stages, the final five combined TNM stages (0–IV), which put all the information together into one final numeric stage bearing prognostic and treatment implications, are often further divided into more substages. Let me give you an example to help you unify all of this staging information floating around in your head. We'll use breast cancer staging for our example. Don't worry if you don't understand the specifics (unless you own a breast cancer, in which case you'll need to learn and understand the specifics through additional reading and by speaking with your physicians). Here we go ...

BREAST CANCER: T STAGE

Stage T0 means that the primary breast tumor cannot be found, but there is breast cancer spread (to the lymph nodes in the armpit and/or to one or more distant sites, such as the lung or liver) proven via biopsy.

97

Stage Tis stands for "carcinoma in situ," a favorable situation in which breast cancer has developed, but the cancer is too small to even be called a tumor and is associated with virtually no chance of spread prior to treatment. These non-tumor cancers are identified on imaging studies (most frequently on mammograms).

Stage T1 tumors are 2cm or less when measured.

Stage T2 tumors are larger than 2cm but less than 5cm when measured.

Stage T3 tumors are larger than 5cm when measured.

Stage T4 tumors may be of any size when measured, but these tumors are growing into (invading) the chest wall (the muscles and/or bone of the chest) and/or the skin overlying the breast.

T Stage Summary: there are six T stages for breast cancer as of today.

BREAST CANCER: N STAGE

Stage N0 cancers have not spread to regional lymph nodes in the axilla (armpit). Strange as this may sound, there are two additional substages for stage N0 breast cancers in which, even though invisible under the microscope (hence N0), cancer cells (called **Stage N0(i+)**) or traces of cancer cells (called **Stage N0(mol+)**) are detected in the regional lymph nodes by special stains or genetic material identification processes.

Stage N1 means that cancer has been found in one to three axillary (armpit) lymph nodes. Stage N1 is further stratified into

Stage N1mi, Stage N1a, Stage N1b, and **Stage N1c** based on measurements and location of the lymph node metastases.

Stage N2 cancers have lymph node mets identified in four to nine axillary lymph nodes or involve another set of non-armpit regional lymph nodes, the internal mammary lymph nodes. N2 includes **Stage N2a and Stage N2b,** based on specific metastasis criteria (we don't need to get into the detailed criteria here).

Stage N3 means even more axillary lymph node mets are found, or metastatic disease has been identified in other non-armpit lymph nodes (associated with a worse prognosis), substaged as **Stage N3a, Stage N3b,** and **Stage N3c** (we don't need to get into the detailed criteria here either).

N Stage Summary: There are four N stages, each further divided into multiple substages . . . complicated!

Breast Cancer: M Stage

Stage M0 means that distant metastatic disease has not been found on any imaging studies or on physical examination. As with N0, there is still an M0 substage, **cM0(i+),** in which cancer cells are identified in the blood or bone marrow or in very tiny deposits in nonregional (distant) lymph nodes.

Stage M1 means that distant metastatic spread has been identified.

M Stage Summary: Fortunately, there are only two main stages, M0 and M1, with clinical meaning for the overwhelming majority of breast cancer patients.

Now we put together all of the differing and complex T, N, and M stages to get a final TNM staging.

BREAST CANCER: OVERALL TNM STAGES

Stage 0 cancers are those staged as **Stage Tis** *and* **Stage N0** *and* **Stage M0** (referred to as **Tis, N0, M0**).

Stage Ia cancers are those staged as **T1, N0, M0.**

Stage Ib cancers are those staged as **T0 or T1, N1mi, M0.**

Stage IIa, Stage IIb, Stage IIIa, Stage IIIb, and **Stage IIIc** get even more complicated, defined by one of several differing combinations of T and N stages (but always with **M0**).

Stage IV (as with all cancers) is defined by one unique thing: **M1** (distant metastatic disease), regardless of T and N stage.

So you can see that TNM staging can get quite complex. And TNM staging (as well as individual T and, for many tumor types, N staging) is unique to each type of cancer. Holy cow! But remember, you only have to understand the TNM staging for your type of cancer. And you do have to understand it, if you are to own it. Read about the specific staging definitions and criteria for your type of cancer on the American Cancer Society website (cancer.org) or other similarly credible websites or publications. And then ask your doctor to explain the many parts of your staging that you will not understand (bring a printout of the website pages with you, having highlighted the areas on which you are unclear). And then ask again. And again. And again, until you understand it. Leave any embarrassment or machismo outside of the physician's office. You simply must get this staging stuff clear in your mind if you are to drive the treatment decisions that will determine your future and your life.

In Practical Terms, How Staging Is Done

Remember that here we're talking about staging your cancer, not diagnosing your cancer. **Diagnosing** is the process of originally determining that you have cancer. Once the presence of cancer anywhere in your body has been proven, the diagnostic process is complete. Some of you were initially diagnosed through non-imaging tests, such as endoscopy (during which a physician looks through a "scope" and can visualize and even biopsy the tissue lining a tubular body structure, such as the bladder, colon, esophagus, stomach, etc.). For the rest of you, imaging studies may have played a role in initially diagnosing your cancer; if so, some or all of those same imaging studies may also be used to determine your N stage and/or your M stage. Regardless of how you were originally diagnosed, imaging studies play the major role in N and M staging, although biopsy may ultimately be required to *prove* the existence of lymph node mets or distant disease. Fortunately, evaluating your regional lymph nodes and searching for distant metastatic disease are two processes that often rely on the same imaging studies. Thus, it is likely that much or all of your N and M staging will be done simultaneously.

For example, the combination of two simple imaging studies, a chest X-ray and a CAT scan of the pelvis and abdomen (both adjacent body regions are rapidly scanned in a single sitting), evaluates the lungs, liver, and lymph nodes—the primary metastatic sites for most cancers, as well as other organs and structures that are less commonly involved with metastases. Thus, for many types of cancer (such as colon, rectal, bladder, prostate, ovarian, uterine, cervix, and others), these two imaging studies may represent all of the testing you undergo to determine both your N and M stage prior to treatment. For certain cancers, particularly those known to frequently metastasize to bone or brain, you may undergo an additional imaging study or two. The addition of blood tests likely completes the M stage evaluation (as I said before, blood tests alone rarely identify metastatic disease). Only if a suspicious growth is identified on one of these imaging studies, or if you have a new physical complaint that requires evaluation, will further imaging studies be performed in search of metastatic disease. Not only do the same studies frequently evaluate your N and M stage simultaneously, for some abdominal or pelvic cancers, the same imaging studies (such as a CAT scan) may even be used to also determine your T stage.

Oh Yeah . . . Staging Can Change

All right. You've learned the basics of staging—no small accomplishment, and critical to owning your cancer. Unfortunately, there's another twist to staging: Staging can change. Your initial cancer stage, before you receive any treatment, is your **clinical stage.** All of the discussion about TNM staging up to now has been about determining your clinical stage. *The clinical stage is what empowers you and your doctors to select the initial treatment that is right both for you and for your cancer.* The clinical stage is like a steak, and selecting your treatment is like grilling that steak. If you haven't ever grilled a steak (and even more so, if you have), at least you've eaten a grilled steak and will therefore understand this comparison (for you vegetarians out there, just play along). If you *undercook* a steak, it's never burned or dry, but it's bloody, soft, and awful, even inedible. If you *overcook* a steak, not only do you create a burnt char on the outside, but the meat is dry, fibrous, tasteless, and awful, even inedible. So, prior to actually grilling a steak, how do I develop my "best guess" in determining all of the elements that go into perfectly grilling (not under- or overcooking) that slab of meat? First, I just look at the steak. I study its size in all three dimensions, paying special attention to how thick it is. I look for the marbling that indicates fat content. I note whether there's a bone coursing through the muscle. Then I throw it on the hot, pre-oiled grill and let the battle begin.

The clinical stage is what empowers you and your doctors to select the initial treatment that is right both for you and for your cancer.

All those things that I do prior to throwing the steak on the grill are part of clinical staging using the TNM system. If grilling represents your cancer treatment (perhaps not the most appealing analogy), then your TNM stage addresses all of my pre-grilling evaluation, because, like your treatment, success in my grilling (a perfectly grilled steak for me; and the best chance of curing your cancer for you) depends on pre-grilling (pre-treatment) knowledge of multiple characteristics (of the steak, for me, and your TNM stage, for you) that directly impact the likelihood of success. How hot should the grill be when I first throw on the meat? When should I turn down the flames? How long should I grill overall? When do I rotate the steak? Flip it? How long should the meat sit after grilling before we eat it? Your treatment considerations are similarly complex and multi-factorial. Whereas undercooking my steak results in a bloody, soft, and awful meal, *your undertreating your cancer reduces your chance of being cured*. Sure, undercooking means no burnt char covering the outside of my steak, just as undertreating your cancer means a lower rate of and less severe treatment side effects and potentially dangerous treatment complications. But again, my undercooked meat is inedible, and your undertreated cancer is still alive and growing. And on the other end of the spectrum? My overcooked meat is dry, firm, and tasteless. And it's burnt to boot. Now, your overtreated cancer has received the treatment required to kill it, and that's priority number one. But overtreating a cancer does not increase your chances of being cured relative to correctly treating your cancer. And like my meat, overtreatment unnecessarily increases your potential to experience awful side effects and dangerous complications. Given that you gain nothing in terms of likely cure from overtreatment, and given that you increase the frequency, intensity, and the risk of unpleasant side effects and serious complications, why would you overtreat your cancer?

Overtreatment unnecessarily increases your potential to experience unpleasant side effects and dangerous complications.

Where were we? Your TNM stage is your clinical stage, which is the best way to determine the initial treatment options most appropriate for you to *correctly* treat your cancer. And unlike my grilling decisions, which are based solely on my own experiences and occasionally on those of my father-in-law (when I'm lucky enough to have him grill-side), the determination of your TNM stage-specific treatment options is based upon information learned from tens and hundreds of thousands of patients with your type of cancer and the experiences of thousands of their physicians. With the exception of clinical trials, which are forms of clinical research required to determine the safety and effectiveness of newly developed treatments (and which we'll discuss in a later chapter), most American physicians who regularly deal with cancer patients are up to speed on stage-specific treatment options; that is, they are master grillers. (We'll have a serious discussion regarding your selection of treatment physicians and treatment center in a later chapter.)

Still, clinical staging is based upon imaging studies and, for some of you, needle biopsies. It's not always correct. So *your clinical stage can change during or following your initial treatment,* replaced by your more accurate **pathological stage.** Pathologic staging takes into account the additional information regarding your cancer that is discovered during treatment, most commonly surgical treatment. For those of you who will not have a surgical procedure included in your treatment strategy, it is likely that your clinical stage will remain as your most up-to-date stage, the "best guess" you'll have regarding your total cancer burden. Another small group of you reading this book will have undergone surgery that provided you with your original cancer diagnosis. For example, I've performed many emergency operations because someone's large bowel was completely obstructed, only to find a colon cancer as the cause of the obstruction. In those cases, I both diagnosed their colon cancer and completed their surgical treatment with that one initial operation. In this situation, there is no clinical stage, just a pathological stage based on the surgical specimens (T and N stages determined by pathologic analysis of the surgically collected tumor and regional lymph nodes), combined with imaging studies soon after surgery to evaluate any distant metastatic disease (M stage). Finally, a very small group of you will not be curable but will undergo surgery to relieve a serious problem caused by your tumor (such as an obstruction or bleeding). But for the majority of you, surgery will serve as the critical, often initial, and occasionally only approach to treating you in an attempt to cure your cancer. Most commonly, surgery is included with other treatments as part of a "multi-modality approach" (we will discuss treatments in an upcoming chapter).

Relative to the preceding clinical stage, the pathological stage has additional, critical information that trumps (supersedes) any conflicting clinical stage conclusions: everything the pathologist finds in the surgical specimen and everything your surgeon found when "exploring" your body at the time of your surgery. The surgical specimen holds vast quantities of relevant information only suggested by or even entirely hidden from the imaging studies used for your initial clinical staging. That specimen includes all the tissue removed by the surgeon: the intact tumor completely encased within a shell of healthy tissue, plus regional lymph nodes, and any adjacent organs, portions of organs, or tissue touched or invaded by your primary tumor. The surgeon's exploration provides additional information, particularly regarding distant metastases small enough to avoid detection, but not hidden from the surgeon's hands or eyes. Many times I have "entered the abdomen" on a colon cancer patient whose clinical image-based staging was "M0" (no distant metastases) only to find unsuspected tiny metastatic tumors spread across the surface of the liver, looking and feeling like large grains of sand strewn across the beach . . . this always makes me so sad.

For many, and hopefully most, of you your surgical findings will have no impact on your disease assessment, and your clinical stage and pathological stage will be the same. Why do I say, "hopefully most of you"? Because a modification of a clinical stage to a *lower* pathological stage (better for you) is uncommon, often resulting from a failure to biopsy a suspicious finding on an imaging study during clinical staging (resulting in Clinical Stage M1) that at surgery is found to not be a met (Pathological Stage M0). For the majority of you whose staging does change following surgery, your pathological stage will be greater (less favorable) than your clinical stage. Why? Think of my example about the "grains of sand" coating the liver that I would discover during surgery but that were not seen on the CAT scan prior to surgery. Small distant metastases can easily go unseen by today's imaging techniques, but these may well be found by the surgeon's hands or eyes, or even by imaging studies used *during* surgery that are much more powerful than those pictures taken prior to surgery. (I routinely apply an ultrasound imaging probe directly to the liver during surgery, greatly enhancing the ability to detect small mets.) More commonly, lymph node metastases too small to be detected by presurgical

CAT scan are found by the pathologist to harbor metastatic cancer cells when the surgical specimen is analyzed.

Finally, even your pathological stage can change, sadly (again) for the worse. If your pathological stage is M0 (no distant metastases) and sometime following treatment distant metastases are identified (a recurrence), your new stage is obviously more advanced (worse) than was your pre-recurrence pathological stage. As we've touched upon, recurrences are the result of metastatic cells already present within the distant site at the time of treatment that were too small (too few in number) to be identified either through imaging studies (clinical staging) or via biopsy (pathological staging). Only with time will these malignant cells replicate to numbers that are visible on a routine follow-up imaging study or of a size that cause pain, blockage, or some other new complaint.

Well, you made it through this, the most difficult chapter. All kidding aside, I'm proud of you. You've invested the time and energy required to gain a basic understanding of the staging of your cancer. Without this knowledge, you can say you do, but you can't really own your cancer. Now you own it, and the next steps are yours.

8

It's All About You, Baby: Picking Your Doctors

There are many things about your cancer that you can't control. For you nonsmokers (and you smokers with a malignancy other than lung cancer), you had no say in your developing cancer (and smokers whose smoking did result in lung cancer ownership need the same help and compassion). And you didn't select from a list the type of cancer you have. The presence or absence of pain, obstruction, or other symptoms was entirely up to the gods. You also had no input into your cancer stage or cell grade when your body decided to grow this thing. While you can (and must) have input regarding your cancer treatment, you don't even get to pick the treatment options (one or more are presented to you, but the options are "picked" by physicians, pharmaceutical and medical equipment companies, the US Food and Drug Administration, and your cancer stage). However, there is one major decision that has enormous potential impact on both your chance of cure and on your quality of life moving forward (even if you are not cured), and it is a decision that many cancer patients leave up to chance or at best, to someone else who doesn't know them well: *which physicians you will partner with* in fighting your malignancy. If you do nothing else as the owner of your cancer, own this process.

There are several facets to picking your cancer doctors. The roles of the surgeon, radiation oncologist, and medical oncologist are quite different, and thus the selection process differs for each. The choice of medical center may also be critical. In this chapter, we will explore these and other issues that you, as the owner of your disease, must understand and on which you must lead the way.

How do most newly diagnosed cancer patients select their doctors? They don't. They're "referred," almost always by their own primary care physician. Thus with little other than the referral of a physician whom they most likely see for no more than fifteen minutes once a year, the newly diagnosed cancer patient accepts without question which physician or physicians will serve as guide and partner on the most important health journey of his or her life. Hell, I'll even watch a movie trailer online before I commit to spending $30 and two hours dragging my family to the theater. *To base such a crucial partnership, a partnership on which your survival literally depends, on the referral of a physician who likely knows little or nothing about you other than that you have cancer (and what you look like in your underwear) is insane.* Is this how you pick your babysitters, and if so, how many children have you lost?

Choosing your doctor has enormous potential impact on both your chance of cure and on your quality of life moving forward (even if you are not cured); if you do nothing else as the owner of your cancer, own this process.

There are several reasons why many of you have already begun traveling down this path. First of all, you were (and may still be) shell-shocked at learning you have cancer. Second of all, what the hell do *you* know about selecting which physician is right for you? Finally, isn't "time of the essence," isn't "the clock ticking"? Let's answer this last question first: The majority of cancers grow and spread at a rate that gives you time to evaluate who and what are the best decisions for you. The cancer that you just learned about a couple of weeks or even months ago is not going to kill you next Thursday. But *choosing the wrong doctor can mean that you have greatly decreased your chance to keep your cancer from killing you some day*. As to the second question, "What the hell do you know about selecting which physician is right for you," the answer is: You will know . . . just keep reading. As to the first question, I know you may still feel shell-shocked . . . get over it. Own this thing and let's get 'er done.

Finding Your Surgeon

Many of you will undergo surgery as part (or even all) of the treatment aimed at curing you. For most of you, surgery will be the initial treatment you receive. You need to understand this: The success of radiation therapy depends to a large extent on the equipment and treatment **protocol** (set of instructions specific for treating your cancer), and the success of chemotherapy depends to a large extent on the pharmaceutical agents (chemotherapy drugs) and treatment protocol; *the success of surgical treatment depends almost entirely on a person: your surgeon.*

Stated differently: Pick a mediocre radiation oncologist or medical oncologist and odds are you'll still receive acceptable treatment; *pick the wrong surgeon and you may dramatically reduce your chance of beating your cancer.* Radiation and chemotherapy depend heavily upon equipment, drugs, and standard guidelines. Surgery depends on a human being. If your surgeon does not have a clear understanding of how to operate on someone with your exact stage of your specific type of cancer, and/or if your surgeon does not have the technical experience and/or skills to perform the surgical procedure most likely to cure you, then what the hell are you doing letting this surgeon care for you? Thus, whether surgery is the initial or sole approach to curing you, or whether your surgery follows radiation and/or chemotherapy in your treatment plan, you'd better pick the right guy or gal to hold the scalpel.

So, how do you know who is the right surgeon for you? There are a number of questions to which you should seek answers. Many can be answered simply by looking on the Internet. Others you may have to ask of the surgeon's staff via a phone call. Still others can only be answered by speaking directly with the surgeon (some of these are summarized in the Appendix at the end of this book). We'll get to these questions in a second, but first, go back and read the title of this chapter. Go ahead . . . I'll wait.

Back? Good. *It's all about you, baby.* That means if you are or were referred to a surgeon by your family doctor of forty years, but you don't like the surgeon's answers to the questions we're about to discuss, *it's too damn bad.* It will hurt your family doctor's feelings if you pass on his referred surgeon? *Too damn bad.* For all you know, the referral is based on the fact that they've golfed together every third Saturday for years (no joke—many physician referrals are based on personal friendships, as most primary care physicians don't clearly know the surgeon's true skills or knowledge). Will it piss off the surgeon that you're going to find someone else to perform your cancer operation? *Too damn bad.* Trust me (I'm a surgeon): The surgeon has a stable ego and he'll/she'll get over it within minutes, if not seconds.

It's all about you, baby. If the surgeon screws up and as a result your cancer recurs (grows back), will it block *your surgeon's* large bowel, will it spread to *your surgeon's* lungs? If the surgeon means well but is inexperienced in dealing with your cancer type or your cancer stage, will your tumor return to fill *your surgeon's* liver full of mets? If the surgeon doesn't do as good a job as possible, will your cancer kill your surgeon . . . or you? It's not about the surgeon. *It's all about you, baby.*

So what makes a good surgeon the right surgeon for you? A good surgeon is

1. interested and experienced in caring for cancer patients

2. interested and experienced in specifically caring for cancer patients with your type of cancer

3. interested and experienced in caring for cancer patients with your type of cancer and your specific stage of cancer

Now understand this: In many surgical fields, there are surgical "generalists" and surgical "specialists." While this differentiation does not always help (we'll discuss that soon), it's not a bad place to start. **Generalist surgeons** (such as general surgeons, gynecologists, head and neck surgeons, orthopedic surgeons, neurosurgeons, and urologists) complete college and medical school, then spend several (usually four to five) years as interns (the first year) and then as surgical residents before heading out to practice surgery. During this training, these future generalist surgeons are required (under supervision) to see, operate on, and care for a wide variety of cancer patients. But there are several factors relating to where they train as residents that impact whether or not they were trained well enough to serve as *your* cancer surgeon. For example, if they were residents at a small, rural hospital, they may not have seen any but the most common cancer types and earliest (least advanced) cancer stages, as patients with less common or more advanced disease were referred elsewhere. So do you need a surgeon trained at a large, inner-city teaching hospital where the really rare and complex cancer cases are also cared for? Perhaps, but sometimes these teaching hospital surgical programs train not only residents but also *surgical fellows*. Surgical fellows have completed their generalist surgical training and chose out of interest to continue with more focused training to become surgical specialists. For example, during my general surgery residency training, my passion for cancer patients led me to spend two additional years in a cancer research lab, and after completing my general surgery residency, I spent an additional year as a colon and rectal surgical fellow focusing solely on the care of patients with intestinal diseases, primarily colorectal cancer. Those surgeons who, like me, complete a fellowship focused on specific types of cancer truly develop additional knowledge, skills, and expertise that can greatly benefit you. Unfortunately for the resident who is training to practice as a surgical generalist, the presence of surgical fellows at the busy training hospital often limits the resident's actual participation in the care of cancer patients (because the fellows are caring for the cancer patients). Thus, at some of the hospitals where I trained as a surgical fellow, the general surgery residents had very little hands-on involvement in the care of the more advanced or unusual intestinal cancer patients. As a result, whether trained in small, rural hospitals or in large, inner-city hospitals with surgical fellows present, some generalist surgeons never really learn how best to deal with many cancer patients. So what to do?

My suggestion is that *if there is a fellowship-trained surgeon available to you* (covered by your insurance and in a location that works for you and your family), *start there*. Of course, the fellowship training had to emphasize *cancer* surgery (it does you no good to see a gynecologic surgeon whose fellowship and expertise are in the area of fertility, or a urologist whose fellowship was focused on kidney transplantation). *Find a surgical specialist whose fellowship training focused heavily on caring for patients with your type of cancer.* Here's a general guide regarding surgical specialists for several types of cancer:

For colon or a rectal cancer, meet with a colon and rectal surgeon. We (I'm one of these guys) specialize in the care of patients who own these two related but in many ways unique large bowel cancers. If there is no fellowship-trained colon and rectal surgeon available (and be careful, as *many general surgeons advertise themselves as colon and rectal surgeons but have not completed fellowship training*, so find out via the Internet or by asking the surgeon directly), you will be in good hands if you find a general surgeon with significant experience and interest in colon or rectal cancer care. One note of warning: *Rectal cancer is very different than colon cancer* and, in my opinion, *should only be treated by a fellowship-trained colon and rectal surgeon* unless impossible for you to find or have covered by your insurer (and don't give up on the latter without a fight). Failure to do so may mean that your rectal cancer is not staged correctly, whereas colon and rectal surgeons (not radiologists) are often the experts in ultrasound staging of your tumor. It may also happen that rectal cancer treatment is not provided in the correct order (some patients benefit from radiation and chemotherapy *prior* to surgery), and surgery may unnecessarily leave you with a permanent colostomy (when the end of the large intestine drains through the wall of your abdomen into a bag).

For pancreatic, hepatic (liver), or biliary (the tubes draining the liver) cancer, meet with either a fellowship-trained surgical oncologist or a fellowship-trained hepatobiliary surgeon. If meeting with the former, make certain that he/she is experienced and interested in the care of patients with your type of cancer. Ask this, because surgical oncologists often focus only briefly on a number of types of cancer during fellowship training, and even after fellowship some still have limited experience with these complicated cancers. If you still cannot find the right surgical specialist, head to an **academic medical center** (a hospital with a medical school, also referred to as a "teaching hospital") and seek out a general surgeon with significant experience and interest in your type of cancer. All major surgical teaching hospitals (that is, those teaching hospitals that train surgery residents) have one or more surgeons who are passionate about the care of pancreatic/hepatic/biliary cancers. Again, do your research—for these types of cancer, search the websites of the academic medical centers nearest you; you will likely find one or more surgeons whose profiles clearly state their interest in these cancers.

For lung cancer, meet with a thoracic (chest) surgeon. Now, this can be tricky, as most thoracic surgeons are actually trained as cardiothoracic surgeons; that is, their fellowship training included heart surgery as well as lung surgery (and the focus on heart surgery is often much greater than the focus on lung cancer). There are only a few pure (no heart) thoracic surgery fellowships that train surgeons who are truly passionate about lung cancer (as well as cancer of the esophagus). That doesn't mean that a cardiothoracic surgeon is not experienced or interested in treating lung cancer; however, many if not most of these surgeons are most passionate about heart surgery. Thus, if no thoracic-only-fellowship-trained surgeon is available to you, find a cardiothoracic surgeon with experience and interest in treating lung cancer. In my opinion, there is no place for a general surgeon in the surgical care of a lung cancer patient.

For esophageal cancer, see the previous bullet on lung cancer, as thoracic (chest) surgeons are also the most experienced and interested in the care of diseases of this thoracic organ. As with lung cancer, if no thoracic-only-fellowship-trained thoracic surgeon is available to you, find a cardiothoracic surgeon with experience and interest in treating esophageal cancer. Unlike with lung cancer, there are a limited number of general surgeons who are experienced and interested in esophageal cancer. That said, this would be my very last choice, and such a general surgeon would have to be practicing at a teaching hospital to provide the required postoperative care.

For cancer of the ovary, uterus, or cervix, seek out a gynecologic oncologist. These are general obstetrician/gynecologists who receive additional fellowship training focused on gynecologic cancers. This is critical, as the vast majority of general obstetrician/gynecologists have very limited training and expertise in the surgical care of gynecologic cancers. In fact, many general obstetrician/gynecologists refer most or all of their gynecologic cancer patients to gynecologic oncologists. Only if no gynecologic oncologist is available (and you should be willing to drive a bit, if necessary) should you seek care from a general obstetrician/gynecologist. If this is your situation, do your homework to make certain that this generalist has significant experience and interest in your cancer type and, especially, stage.

For prostate cancer (which rarely needs surgery), bladder cancer, or renal (kidney) cancer, you should see a urologist. You should not be overly concerned if you can't find a fellowship-trained urologist whose fellowship focused on cancer, both because this is very uncommon and because many general urologists have significant experience in the surgical treatment of these cancers. That said, many urologists focus on benign conditions, like prostatic hypertrophy (enlarged prostate), erectile dysfunction, and urinary incontinence (involuntary urine loss). Again, find the urologist who not only has experience but also clearly has real interest in your type and stage of cancer.

The approach to surgeon selection is the same for cancers not mentioned on this list: If there is a surgeon who has completed not only general surgical training but also additional fellowship training with some or complete focus on your type of cancer, that surgeon's office is a good first place to visit. If not, thoroughly research the generalist surgeons available to you. Look on the surgeon's Internet site, as physicians routinely present their areas of professional expertise and interest. Don't be shy about calling the surgeon's office and speaking with the surgeon's nurse (remember, it's all about you, baby, so who cares about a little embarrassment when you're trying to get cured). Ask about the surgeon's experience regarding your type and stage of cancer. And if the previous steps lead you to the generalist surgeon's office for an introductory meeting, own your cancer, step up, and ask specifically about that surgeon's experience (training, number of patients routinely cared for, outcomes, complications, and other questions detailed in the Appendix at the end of this book) in treating cancer patients with your type of cancer and your stage of cancer. Don't be shy, don't feel embarrassed or guilty, and don't be afraid to ask questions and seek answers. It's all about you, baby.

You may well ask if you should look for a surgical specialist who has completed both general surgical and subsequent fellowship training regardless of your cancer type or stage. The answer is yes, but the reality is that there are not enough fellowship-trained surgical specialists to care for every cancer patient. In addition, specialist surgeons tend to cluster around teaching hospitals and larger cities where there are enough cancer patients to support their focused practices. That's why today most surgery performed on cancer patients is performed by generalist surgeons. Don't worry . . . there are many tremendous generalist surgeons out there who can provide you with high-quality, compassionate care. And understand this: Some generalist surgeons are passionate about cancer patients and focus much or all of their practices on the treatment of one or a few types of cancers. Breast cancer is such an example. General surgeons are all trained in the basic care of breast cancer patients, and most practice breast cancer surgery on a regular basis. Given how few fellowship-trained surgical oncologists are out there (who have received additional knowledge, skills, and expertise in the treatment of cancer of the breast, among other cancers), the majority of breast cancer surgery is performed—and performed quite well—by general surgeons. But remember, *there is a big difference between a general surgeon who operates on a breast cancer patient every few weeks or months and a general surgeon who operates on several breast cancer patients weekly or even every day*. A general surgeon who has made the personal and professional commitment to heavily focus his or her career on breast cancer frequently becomes as knowledgeable and skilled in breast cancer care as a fellowship-trained specialist, as she or he constantly reads about new treatments, techniques, and information regarding the disease and attends meetings and courses focused on breast cancer. However, again, if a fellowship-trained surgical specialist is available, start there.

Finding Your Radiation Oncologist

As I emphasized in the beginning of this chapter, no one physician selection is as critical as your choice (*your* choice) of surgeon. For those of you who will undergo radiation therapy, your selection of your radiation oncologist is also important, but your overall success in receiving the best possible radiation therapy (treatment) for your type and stage of cancer is much less reliant on this individual doctor. This is because your surgeon has to have knowledge, experience, and significant technical skills to best assist you in achieving a cure. Your radiation oncologist, on the other hand, has to possess only the first two of these qualities, and the first is truly the most important. That is, your "rad onc" must be knowledgeable in the treatment of your type and stage of cancer. While experience does matter, unlike surgery (where experience is a must), the rad onc does not himself or herself deliver the radiation treatment to you. Radiation is delivered either by large pieces of external equipment or through the temporary implantation of small radiation-emitting pellets; either way, the radiation therapy is based on a complex treatment plan designed specifically for you by your rad onc, a physicist, and radiation technologists. Your radiation doses (called "fractions") and the delivery of these fractions are based on a treatment protocol: guidelines provided by expert radiation oncology societies, top academic medical centers, and recognized radiation oncologist leaders, all of which are available to your doctor through his or her training and continuing education (such as meetings, journals, and lectures). Thus the vast majority of radiation oncologists are competent in planning your radiation treatment, which is then delivered to you by advanced equipment or radiation implants, with the input of the physicist and radiation technologists. That said, you should certainly research the individual rad onc physicians you are considering via the Internet, through queries to the office staff (nurses and radiation technologists), and by directly questioning and speaking with the physician candidates (again, see the Appendix at the end of

There is a critical factor to consider when you select your radiation physician: the radiation delivery system. this book for suggested questions to ask). Repeat the mantra with me: "I won't be shy, won't feel embarrassed or guilty, and won't be afraid to ask questions and seek answers." *It's all about you, baby.*

While the majority of radiation oncologists can deal with the majority of cancer types and stages, there is a critical factor to consider when you select your radiation physician: *the radiation delivery system.* Today's commercial radiation therapy equipment and delivery techniques are big business. Thus, large and small radiation oncology equipment companies are constantly inventing new technologies and techniques to irradiate cancers, all aimed at reducing the complications associated with radiation therapy, increasing the usefulness of radiation therapy, and shortening overall treatment requirements. The pace at which this technological evolution is occurring is staggering. Today there are a variety of new, proven, FDA-approved radiation delivery systems to treat a variety of cancers, such as breast and lung cancer. These new modalities may provide you a safer radiation treatment without sacrificing the likelihood of successfully killing your cancer. In addition, some of these advances demand fewer total treatments, shortening your radiation therapy program—a real logistical benefit for you and your family, who will frequently be driving you back and forth for several weeks.

But such cutting-edge technology can only help you if your radiation oncologist has the newer technology and uses it. Thus, *own your cancer and ask what equipment and approach the rad onc would recommend specifically for you.* Many times physicians who don't own or have access to the newest technology (often because of the incredible cost) will assure you that the new stuff is "no better than what we use." Now, that may be true, but if not (more likely), move on, even if you like the physician. After all, you wouldn't eat in a restaurant with lousy food simply because you like the chef, would you? Then again, sometimes the new technology *is* no better than what they use. So how can you tell the value of new technology? Again, a little research goes a long, long way. And since you own your cancer, you have accepted the responsibility to learn as best you can so that you can lead the decision-making processes aimed at saving your life. *New technology that is truly better is often first routinely used by nationally recognized cancer centers.* Thus, read about the radiation equipment and approaches used to treat your specific cancer type and stage on the website of major, credible cancer centers (I list many such renowned cancer centers and their web addresses in Chapter 3 and in the Resources section at the end of this book). Understand that you don't have to receive your radiation therapy at one of these legendary institutions (although if you can, you won't be sorry); you're simply trying to determine what equipment and approach these radiation therapy experts have themselves selected for use in treating patients like you. If they believe that a newer technology and/or technique is best for their cancer patients, shouldn't you receive the same treatment? If an older treatment technique seems to still be the accepted approach at these centers, then it's reasonable that the rad onc with whom you met also wouldn't treat you with the "newest and greatest" gadget. Whichever the case, you'll find out through your research efforts what is being utilized at these top-tier institutions and then find a rad onc just down the street (and covered by your insurance) who will offer you the same radiation treatment approach (it's like having the greatest Chinese food in New York delivered right to your home in Billings).

Finding Your Medical Oncologist

A medical oncologist is the physician who recommends chemotherapy drug options to you and, once a treatment is selected, calculates how best to deliver the drugs to you (dose you). Now they may not like my next statement, but the medical oncologist is far and away the easiest of your new three-physician team to select. You know that selecting your surgeon largely comes down to, "Does this doctor know what to do, and does he/she have the technical skills to adequately perform the right cancer operation?" Finding your radiation oncologist is much less perilous, as the question is, "Does this doctor know what to do or, if not, can he/she read what to do, and does he/she have the right equipment?" For the medical oncologist (most often simply referred to as the oncologist), the question is even shorter and simpler: "Does this doctor know what to do or, if not, can he/she read what to do?" That's because the oncologist (like the radiation oncologist and unlike the surgeon) does not utilize technical skill in treating you. In fact, your oncologist could call in the drug orders from a bathtub on a cruise ship and it wouldn't negatively impact the success of your chemotherapy treatment. Nor does the oncologist depend on expensive equipment to deliver your treatment (unlike the radiation oncologist). The oncologist relies solely on the knowledge—either personal or attainable—of what **drug regimen** (group of chemotherapy drugs) you should receive, how to calculate your dose (that is, how much you should receive, how often, and for how long), and, if necessary, how to address side effects and complications that develop. Unlike radiation oncology equipment, every oncologist pretty much has access to every approved chemotherapy drug (or an equivalent) that you might need. And the drugs are administered either during out-patient visits to his/her office (after which you go home) through an intravenous (IV) line, by you at your home (you swallow pills), or, rarely, during brief hospitalizations. So the critical thing is that you are presented with the most recently approved best therapies. This is usually the case, but sometimes in smaller communities, and with older oncologists, this may not be so. How do you know? You own your cancer, so remember what I've just taught you about selecting your surgeon and your radiation oncologist: *The best new chemotherapeutic regimens (treatments) are often first adopted for use by nationally recognized cancer centers.* Thus, read about the medical oncology (chemotherapy) approach used to treat your specific cancer type and stage on the website of a major cancer center (again, I refer you to the brilliant and engaging Chapter 3 and Resources section). And again, just as with radiation therapy, you don't have to be treated at one of these legendary institutions (although if you can be, you won't be sorry). You're simply trying to determine what these chemotherapy experts have themselves selected for use in treating patients specifically like you. If the patients at the great cancer centers are receiving a specific chemotherapeutic treatment, shouldn't you?

There is one unique aspect that distinguishes your relationship with the oncologist from your relationship with either the surgeon or rad onc: For most of you, your oncologist will be the cancer physician with whom you spend the greatest time during treatment and likely the main (or even sole) physician with whom you regularly engage in the many years of post-treatment follow-up surveillance for cancer recurrence. In other words, this is the man/woman with whom you will have the tightest and longest relationship, so make sure that you like the person wearing the white coat. Many oncologists tend to be cynical and even outwardly depressed (understandable, given what they deal with on a daily basis). Others are upbeat and optimistic. And most, in my experience, fall in between, responding differently to each patient's personality. Find someone who seems the best fit for you.

And just one side note: While selecting your medical oncologist may be the easiest of your three physician choices, oncologists are, in general, the smartest docs in the cancer world. The vast repository of chemotherapy drug and treatment outcome data stored within the average oncologist's brain never ceases to amaze a simple surgeon like me. If when meeting an oncologist you are not blown away by how much they know, the facts and figures that he/she can pull out in a fraction of a second, then leave that physician's office immediately. They are, put simply, brainiacs.

Going to a Major Cancer Center

I've referred a number of times to world-renowned, leading cancer centers. I've been blessed to have worked as a surgeon in such centers, and I am a true believer. But I'm also a realist. Your access is likely restricted by your health-care insurance guidelines. And/ or you may be restricted by your personal finances. And/or you may not live anywhere near such a famed institution. And even if you can afford to travel far away to receive your care at such a center, you and your family may not wish to or be able to be apart during your treatment. So here's the deal: If you follow these simple guidelines, you'll sacrifice little or nothing if, for any of the reasons I've just mentioned or for any of a dozen more, you cannot receive your treatment from a top-tier cancer center:

- As discussed, you don't need to go to a leading cancer center to receive the best chemotherapy for you. Any competent medical oncologist has access to the identical proven and approved protocols (instructions and guidelines), as well as to the exact same proven and approved chemotherapy drugs that they use at the Mayo Clinic and elsewhere. It doesn't matter if the drugs are given to you in the back of your oncologist's old Chevy, as long as you make certain that you are offered the same treatment regimen that the big boys are using.

- Also as discussed, the same holds true for your radiation therapy. Just confirm that the technology and approach being used to deliver your radiation are the same as you'd receive at a leading cancer center.

- While a nationally recognized cancer center will no doubt deliver a surgical specialist with the experience, interest in, and passion for treating your type and stage of cancer, similar surgeons are also found at lesser known medical centers, particularly (teaching) academic centers. Thus, if there is a teaching hospital that trains surgical residents near you (particularly one associated with a university), first try finding your surgeon there. If not, there are appropriately competent surgeons at many larger community hospitals. And remember, even if you have to travel quite a distance, unlike radiation and chemotherapy, surgery is a one-time, short-term venture. Thus, you can be far from home for a couple of weeks if it means that you are being cared for by the surgeon who gives you the greatest chance of achieving a cure.

- And remember: There is no rule that says your surgeon, radiation oncologist, and/or medical oncologist all have to work at the same place. As a colon and rectal cancer expert at a respected cancer center, it was not uncommon for me to meet patients who had traveled great distances to have me perform their cancer operations. Their radiation therapy was performed elsewhere, closer to home, as was their chemotherapy (re-read the last two sentences of the previous bullet regarding surgery).

One final note: All of the best cancer centers, the overwhelming majority of teaching hospitals, and a significant number of community hospitals that care for numerous cancer patients utilize an organized structure called a **Tumor Board.** Tumor Boards are made up of surgeons, radiation oncologists, medical oncologists,

There is no rule that says your surgeon, radiation oncologist, and/or medical oncologist all have to work at the same place.

and (on the better Tumor Boards) radiologists and pathologists, all of whom have experience with, interest in, and a passion for treating cancer patients. The role of the Tumor Board is to develop a single consensus recommendation regarding treatment (and sometimes staging) that is specific to you as an individual cancer patient. Thus, the Tumor Board not only considers what type and stage of cancer you own, the Board also considers your individual health status (other medical conditions, medications you are taking, your age, whether you smoke, etc.). By representing a broad spectrum of cancer doctors, no one physician's treatment bias drives your treatment recommendation, and you gain from an exponential amount of combined knowledge and experience rather than just relying on the experiences and bias of a single physician. While not necessarily a reason to reject a physician or facility, the absence of a Tumor Board should give you pause . . . and make you consider seeking other options.

For many of you, while the title and main message of this chapter is easy to understand and agree with ("put all emotions and social norms aside and do what is best for you"), translating this critical concept into actions, *your actions*, will be challenging. You are thoughtful and polite (you're obviously not a surgeon). You avoid both embarrassing yourself and insulting others (again, clearly not a surgeon). You don't challenge others, especially "experts," and least of all doctors. You do not regularly *lead* activities or decisions, especially not activities or decisions for which the stakes are so high and your knowledge and experience so limited. For you, it will be an enormous challenge to abandon many of these wonderful qualities that have guided you through your whole life up to now, allowing you to be loved by friends and colleagues alike. But you must be aggressive in personally selecting your physician partners. Failure to put aside these parts of who you are, failure to take on this critical responsibility of cancer ownership, may lead to catastrophic results. After all, what's the use of being such a wonderful human being, father, mother, husband, wife, friend . . . if you're not around? Own your cancer and remember: *It's all about you, baby.*

9

The Witches' Brew:
Understanding Cancer Treatments

The thickest chapter in most cancer textbooks is the one discussing cancer treatments. Why so many pages? Because every type of cancer and every stage of every type of cancer is treated in a unique way. To further complicate matters, there are often multiple treatment options for the same cancer type and stage. Why? There's a saying in surgery:

If there's more than one way to do something, then there's no one best way.

There are often many options for treatment of the same cancer because, as complex as many cancer treatment strategies are, no one treatment regimen (mixture of treatments) proves to be significantly better than the others. Thus, several treatment regimens may have similar cure rates, but each treatment regimen has its own "toxicity profile" (this one makes you throw up, that one risks lung injury, and the other one can damage your pancreas). Some treatments are not used for people with liver disease; others must be avoided by those with compromised kidney function. It truly is overwhelmingly complex.

This chapter on understanding cancer treatments will not be as long as similar chapters found in most cancer textbooks. We will not be discussing specific treatments for each and every type and stage of cancer (specific surgical procedures, individual chemotherapy drug combinations, etc.). No. But this will be the thickest chapter in *this* book. We will be discussing many important general concepts regarding the varying types of treatments and approaches that you'll need to understand and consider when making treatment decisions, because while you cannot impact what treatment options you are offered (that's up to the FDA, pharmaceutical companies, physicians, and others), as the owner of your cancer, you and you alone will have to choose which if any of the recommended treatment options you will receive.

As the owner of your cancer, you and you alone should choose which if any of the recommended treatment options you will receive.

The Lowdown on "The Big Three"

The general local-regional-distant approach to mapping out your cancer is also useful in understanding the roles that surgery, radiation therapy, and chemotherapy ("The Big Three") play in cancer treatment. By definition, for you to achieve a "cure," every living cancer cell in your body must be destroyed, as any remaining cancer will multiply and grow, finally being identified as a cancer recurrence. The Big Three each play primary and secondary roles in eradicating all the cancer that is known or suspected (based on your tumor type and stage) to be living within your body.

Surgery: First Among Equals

Remember in the last chapter how I separated the impact of your choice of surgeon from the impact of your choice of radiation oncologist and medical oncologist? There is a related separation of surgical treatment from all nonsurgical treatments that is simple to understand but should not be underappreciated. Here goes. Once you're in the operating room and the anesthesiologist puts you to sleep, *you have no further say in your surgical treatment.* You'll be asleep when critical decisions regarding your cancer surgery and your quality of life are being made (such as how much normal tissue surrounding the tumor should be removed; what should be done if there is an unexpected finding of a metastasis; should an operation leave you with a permanent colostomy and stool collection bag on your abdomen when the need for such an outcome wasn't anticipated; should you be kept alive by lifesaving intervention if something goes wrong; and so on and so on and so on). *Your surgeon alone will be continuously making decisions that dramatically impact not only your chance of cure but also your quality of life following surgery.* Get it? Once you say, "Nighty-night," it's all in the hands of your surgeon—and that's a very big "all." This is why, as the owner of your cancer, you must find the surgeon who is experienced, interested, caring, and right for you. This is why, as the owner of your cancer, you should discuss potentially important intraoperative decisions and life-impacting outcomes with your surgeon prior to undergoing surgery, such as your feelings about life-sustaining efforts (discussed in Chapter 10). A surgeon who strongly disagrees with your desires regarding such critical decisions should not remain your surgeon, but you won't know this until you have the conversation.

The primary role of surgery is to completely resect (remove) your *local* disease (primary tumor). If you have breast cancer, surgery will likely be recommended to remove the primary tumor. Stomach cancer? Surgery will likely be recommended to remove some or all of your stomach. Colon or rectum? Same thing. While surgery only rarely plays a role in the treatment of some types of cancer (some lung cancers, lymphomas and leukemias, anal cancer, and a handful of others), *surgery routinely is required for most cancers if you are to have a shot at being cured.*

> *As the owner of your cancer, you must discuss potentially important intra-operative decisions and life-impacting outcomes with your surgeon prior to undergoing surgery.*

In removing your primary tumor, the surgeon will do everything he/she can to avoid cutting into or across the cancer, as this can spill cancer cells into your body (you guessed it . . . a bad thing). In fact, the surgeon will not even "carve out" your tumor from the surrounding normal tissues. Why? Because when a pathologist looks under the microscope at a carved-out cancer, cancer cells are frequently visible at the edge of the surgical specimen. This suggests a high likelihood that invisible deposits of living cancer cells were left behind during surgery, surviving to grow into a recurrent cancer. *The best chance at curing you, and the standard of care in cancer surgery, is to remove your tumor encased within a thick rim of normal (non-malignant) tissue.* This means that you may have to sacrifice healthy, functioning tissue structures that you'd rather not lose. For example, if a stomach cancer is growing up against your intestine, rather than "peeling" the tumor off the intestine (which will likely leave stomach cancer cells to grow on the outside of the intestine), your surgeon will remove the stomach cancer, including much or all of your normal stomach, with a portion of normal abutting intestine attached. Surgery must eradicate all local disease by removing your tumor within and attached to surrounding, seemingly normal tissue structures, all in one piece. Where this gets less than black-and-white, and where you'll need to speak about your wishes with your surgeon prior to surgery, is when removing your cancer within a shell of healthy tissue may mean removing an important nerve (to your leg, for example) or important structure (your ovary) in order to completely remove your primary cancer and potentially cure you. *Don't leave such decisions up to anyone other than you.*

While the first role of surgery in the treatment of cancer is to remove (resect) your primary tumor (treating your *local* disease), there is an additional primary role for surgical treatment: *regional* disease resection. During the surgical resection of your primary tumor, your surgeon will also remove the surrounding tissues to collect a large number of the regional lymph nodes that have been draining lymphatic fluid (and, potentially, traveling cancer cells) from your primary tumor. Whether removing any lymph node metastases is itself beneficial in the actual treatment of your cancer is controversial (some physicians believe that these small cancer cell deposits would be destroyed by subsequent chemotherapy and/or radiation if not removed surgically), everyone agrees that the surgical removal of the regional lymph nodes is absolutely necessary to adequately provide you with an accurate pathological stage. It is, unfortunately, not uncommon for patients pre-operatively clinically staged as N0 (no evidence of lymph node mets) to have cancer identified in their regional lymph nodes when the pathologist examines the surgical specimen (thus increasing their clinical stage to a higher, less favorable, pathological stage). But think of it this way: While the unanticipated finding of "positive" lymph nodes in the surgical specimen does increase your stage, the result of this stage correction is *providing you a better chance at curing your now–accurately staged cancer.*

Something else important to appreciate about the surgical removal of your regional lymph nodes: *Which and how many lymph nodes the surgeon must remove is specific to your type of cancer.* So, again, it is critical that you select the right surgeon to treat your cancer. For example, not that long ago breast cancer patients had all of the lymph nodes in their axilla (armpit) on the side of their tumor removed by the surgeon and analyzed by a pathologist for staging. This extensive lymph node resection risked damaging important nerves and permanently leaving the patients with arms that would repeatedly swell and develop infections. Then a series of clinical trials demonstrated that lymph fluid flowed in a predictable pattern from a breast cancer through the lymph nodes under the arm. This allowed for a technique widely utilized today (which, if you are a breast cancer patient, will probably be used if you select the right surgeon) in which a dye is injected *during surgery* into the breast tissue adjacent to the tumor. The injected dye rapidly enters the lymphatic vessels, highlighting the lymphatic journey that a metastatic breast cancer cell would likely take. The dye is identified as it collects within the first lymph node along its journey, called the *sentinel node*. The surgeon easily identifies and removes this first lymph node (the sentinel node) and immediately sends it to the pathologist while the patient remains asleep in the operating room. The pathologist immediately examines the sentinel node for evidence of any metastatic breast cancer, calling the results into the operating room. If the sentinel node is negative (no metastatic breast cancer cells), the surgeon leaves the remaining lymph nodes alone, and the patient avoids the significant complications risked with the older "take all the nodes out" strategy. If the sentinel node is positive, the remaining lymph nodes may be removed to complete pathologic staging (as different lymph node met numbers and patterns require different treatments), but at least the patient is risking complications based on real results and for the right reason, to accurately stage and determine the most appropriate treatment and prognosis for her cancer. Colon and rectal cancers are entirely different than breast cancer. Studies have shown that a minimum of twelve regional lymph nodes must be removed to make a correct determination of pathological stage (this is a statistical, not clinical, numerical requirement). Therefore, surgical removal of fewer than twelve regional lymph nodes is a failure to perform the correct colon or rectal cancer operation. These are examples of the second primary role of surgery: to remove regional lymph nodes for accurate pathological staging.

Finally, in a small group of patients, surgery is also used to treat *distant* disease, either in an attempt to achieve that rare cure of metastatic disease (such as resecting a small number of liver metastases in a colon cancer patient) or as **palliation,** which is not aimed at cure but seeks only to reduce a patient's symptoms (for example, removal of a tumor that is bleeding or blocking the intestine), both of which we will touch on later in this chapter. Overall, it is most appropriate and simplest to think of surgery as the best treatment of your local disease (primary tumor) and the means of simultaneously providing regional lymph nodes for accurate pathological staging.

So how do you know what is the best surgical treatment for you, the operation that will give you the greatest chance of ultimately being cured? Good question. When it comes to surgery, if you have a common type of cancer, there often is only one surgical procedure recommended and used across the country. For example, if you have a cancer within your right colon (large intestine) and have no evidence of distant metastases, every competent surgeon will perform the same operative procedure, removing the same portion of your colon. Notice I said "competent." Because while removing the same portion of the colon is something every surgeon is taught, if you select a surgeon with limited experience and interest in colon cancer, he or she may fail to remove the twelve or more regional lymph nodes required by the pathologist to correctly stage you, increasing the guesswork in recommending postoperative treatment for you. Yet again, *it's about picking the right surgeon*. But my point here is that frequently only one operation is universally recommended. There may be subtle differences, some of which are worth discussing, but for the most part, experienced, interested cancer surgeons all basically perform similar cancer operations for common types and stages of malignancies.

What you do need to discuss with your surgeon are the basic details of the planned operation, the risks relating to the procedure (both short-term and long-term), the most likely important decisions that will need to be made during the operation (while you're asleep), the anticipated duration and challenges associated with your recovery, and how your surgery fits within the time line of your overall treatment (unless, of course, surgery is your only treatment).

Radiation Therapy: Frying Your Nodes Off

Unlike during surgery, when undergoing radiation therapy, you are awake and able to interact with your caregivers. Thus, if you need to stop your radiation therapy during your weeks or months of treatment you can, although it's extremely rare to find radiation side effects intolerable or to have to make critical lifesaving or quality-of-life decisions during radiation treatment. However, you should always feel empowered to discuss any treatment side effects (fatigue, "sunburn," etc.) with your radiation oncologist, as there may be options to help reduce them. And if you should find yourself truly suffering, you should immediately call your rad onc, as rarely, serious complications can indeed develop (and should not "wait until morning").

Radiation therapy is sort of like surgery in reverse, when it comes to its goals. The number-one role for radiation therapy is *regional* treatment. Thus, when lymph node metastases are identified within the surgical specimen, post-surgery radiation therapy is the main weapon used to "sterilize" any remaining regional lymph nodes (to hopefully destroy any malignant cells living within regional lymph nodes that were not removed by the surgeon, as the surgeon neither tries nor would easily be able to remove every lymph node in the region). Thus, the finding of lymph node mets in the surgical specimen indicates the significant potential that there are cancer cells within the remaining regional nodes. Radiation is also used post-operatively for some cancers, such as breast cancer, to destroy microscopic clusters of malignant cells that are potentially left in the non-lymphatic regional tissue following surgical removal of the primary tumor. So radiation is primarily used for *regional* disease treatment. However, a second (and much less common) primary use of radiation therapy is when there is evidence of remaining *local* disease (again, the two primary roles are reversed from those of surgery). Sometimes the surgeon simply cannot remove the entire primary tumor, as doing so would either kill or permanently and significantly injure the patient. In such cases (and believe me as a surgeon, leaving behind "gross tumor" is a sickening feeling), the surgeon knows at the end of the operation that you will need radiation treatment targeting the *local* site in an attempt to kill all of the primary tumor he/she had to leave behind. In other patients, the surgeon removes all gross (visible) tumor, but the pathologist identifies microscopic groups of cancer cells very near or at the surgical margin. The pathologist can only conclude that some microscopic primary tumor cells were left behind following surgery. In both of these scenarios, radiation therapy is used following the patient's recovery from surgery to "bat cleanup" in an attempt to kill any viable cancer cells remaining postoperatively at the local primary tumor site. Finally, as with surgery, radiation is occasionally used as palliative treatment to treat pain or other local, regional, and/or distant metastatic complications in a patient who is not curable. Fortunately, painful bone mets and some other miserable metastatic symptoms are often quite responsive to palliative radiation.

So how do you know what radiation treatment is best for you, which approach is most likely to help cure you of your disease? Radiation therapy is only slightly more complex than surgery when it comes to treatment options. As mentioned in the previous chapter on physician selection, the real question to ask regarding radiation therapy is whether your doctor utilizes the most appropriate equipment and technique for your type and stage of cancer. As we discussed, this is not always the newest available treatment, but it may well be. Remember, your goal is to use the most advanced proven therapy with the fewest side effects and, if possible, the shortest and/or easiest therapy schedule.

Chemotherapy: Clear as (Toxic) Mud

Unlike surgery, when you are receiving chemotherapy, you are awake, alert, and can interact with your oncologist. Also unlike surgery, "chemo" is not a one-time event. It consists of many, many repetitive treatments often administered over many, many months. So you must continue to be actively involved in the assessment and decisions regarding your chemo during treatment. Much more so than with radiation therapy, the potential side effects and serious complications resulting from chemotherapy administration may be severe, so *you must always feel empowered to discuss how you're doing openly and honestly (and immediately, regardless of time of day) with your oncologist*. It's important for you to know that it is extremely common for more than one chemo drug to be given during treatment; a chemotherapy "regimen" is a combination of chemotherapeutic drugs used to treat a single patient, all with their own side effects. Let's say that you begin your chemotherapy treatment regimen by receiving intravenous (IV) drugs in your oncologist's office. Within a couple of days, just as your doctor expected, you're more nauseated than you've ever been. A couple of (very long) days later, you feel exhausted but much better, no longer nauseated, but weakened by your first chemo experience. Next thing you know, you're back in the chemo bay (the room in which you sit while receiving your drugs), and the nausea war begins anew. This is not an uncommon scenario for cancer owners. For many, the post-chemo nausea lessens over time, as their body seemingly gets used to the toxic agents. But let's say that you're one of those unfortunates for whom the nausea doesn't improve, and you've got dozens of chemo treatments ahead of you. Because this is nonsurgical treatment, you are awake during and between the months of chemo treatments, and so you can talk with your oncologist, your family, your friends, whomever. Because as the owner of your cancer, you can demand a change in your treatment or even permanently stop your chemotherapy treatment whenever you choose to do so. Understand? Now, also understand this: *I do not recommend, let alone encourage, that you stop receiving your chemotherapy*. But for those of you who truly cannot tolerate the side effects of your chemotherapy regimen, I do recommend and encourage you to talk openly and honestly with your oncologist. Your doctor may not be aware of how much of a struggle you're having *unless you tell her/him*, and she/he may be able to provide you with medications that reduce the nastiness caused by your chemotherapy agents. Your doctor may also be able to adjust your treatment (the dosage and/or administration schedule) to try to make your chemo more tolerable. And should all else fail and you decide that enough is enough, your oncologist may be able to offer an alternative treatment regimen that for you results in fewer and less severe side effects.

Again, please don't get me wrong. I do not recommend that you bail on your chemotherapy treatment unless you are truly in the very small minority of patients who cannot survive the limited months of treatment despite all of your oncologist's best efforts to reduce the intolerable side effects. But for the overwhelming majority of cancer patients, *it is empowering to simply recognize that you own your cancer and, therefore, you can openly complain to your oncologist about any chemo side effects and demand assistance and, ultimately, even choose to terminate your treatment.*

You must always feel empowered to discuss how you're doing openly and honestly (and immediately, regardless of time of day) with your oncologist.

Unlike surgery or radiation therapy, chemo travels throughout your body. Thus, chemotherapy is the only one of The Big Three treatments that is primarily used to treat known or suspected distant metastatic disease. Circulating throughout your bloodstream, these toxic drugs have one goal and one goal only: to kill each and every cancer cell that is hiding within your body. In general terms, chemotherapy is poison that is especially targeted to kill your particular type of cancer cells. In reality, these highly toxic drugs do not only target cancer cells, and normal cells and tissues are frequently damaged by the chemo as it travels throughout the body. Some organs and tissues are relatively resistant to these toxic, circulating agents (and, therefore, reasonably unaffected), while other organs and tissues are highly sensitive, resulting in side effects such as nausea, hair loss, and diarrhea, and even the potential for significant complications such as impaired liver function and reduced immune function to fight off infections. Pharmaceutical companies are constantly striving to develop better and better agents, defined as chemo drugs that are more toxic to cancer cells and/or less toxic to normal tissues.

Chemotherapy enters your bloodstream either directly, when administered into your vein, or soon after you swallow a chemo pill or liquid. As I said, once in your circulatory system, chemo goes almost everywhere in your body. There are, however, a handful of tissues where it is difficult to accumulate a high enough chemo drug concentration to effectively kill a cancer. For those malignancies, other, non–circulatory system routes are used to deliver chemotherapy. For example, tumors of the central nervous system (spine and brain) may be treated by direct chemotherapy injection into the cerebrospinal fluid that bathes these critical structures. For other tumors, a non-bloodstream route may mean few or no side effects for the cancer owner while still blasting the malignant cells. Bladder cancer is one such cancer, and chemotherapy may be administered via instillation of chemo agents directly into the bladder through a catheter. And there are a few other cancers for which bloodstream-based chemotherapy is not used. However, for the overwhelming majority of you who will receive chemo, you will be receiving the drugs either directly or indirectly into your bloodstream.

Since chemotherapy's primary target is distant metastatic disease, it is obviously administered to patients who have distant mets identified during their initial staging (Clinical Stage M1) or subsequent postoperative staging (Pathological Stage M1). But chemo is most frequently used in M0 (no evidence of distant mets) patients with malignant cells identified within their surgically removed regional lymph nodes (Pathological Stage N1 or greater). Remember: Regional lymph node spread is also evidence that your primary tumor has successfully metastasized, so even if cancer is found in only a single of many surgically removed regional lymph nodes, you'll most likely need chemo to maximize your chance of cure. Let's put it this way. If you live in Florida, as I do, you have to think about snakes. A lot. So if my wife, my two daughters, and I each leave a pair of shoes overnight in the yard, and if in the morning I find a coral snake (you remember . . . "Red on yellow, kill a fellow") in one of my shoes, but if we find no snake in my other shoe or either of my wife's shoes, do you honestly think we'll allow our daughters to slip their feet into their shoes without first checking for snakes? Same with a metastatic lymph node. Finding just one regional lymph node harboring cancer cells is all you need to get your ticket punched to chemo island, even if a bunch of other nodes are cancer-free. Get it? Pretty much any lymph node metastasis demonstrates that your cancer has real metastatic potential and that you may have malignant cells still hiding in your body, meaning you get chemo.

Up to now, the chemo story should make sense: If you have proven distant metastatic disease (called gross metastatic disease, because it is non-microscopic and "grossly" identifiable on imaging studies or by the surgeon) or if you have proven microscopic regional lymph node mets, chemotherapy will almost certainly be recommended. But there are also a few types of cancer for which, even in the absence of distant mets (M0) and regional lymph node mets (N0), chemotherapy is strongly recommended. For these selected N0M0 cancers, decades of experience representing tens and hundreds of thousands of patients have demonstrated that there is a high likelihood that microscopic metastases are hiding somewhere within the patient's body regardless of their N0M0 staging (especially within the liver and/or lung). Therefore, chemo is recommended to these patients based solely upon the known very high metastatic potential of their cancers despite the absence of proven gross distant or microscopic regional metastatic disease. With these very few types of cancer (some sarcomas, for example), we simply *know* from the extensive published medical reports that you very likely already harbor micro-metastatic distant disease that is simply too small to detect. Without chemo, those micro-mets will grow, and your chance of survival will shrink.

One quick general comment. Since chemo is "cancer poison," why limit its use to metastatic disease? Why not use chemo to kill the primary tumor as well, avoiding surgery and the associated surgical risks? A cynic would say that such a solution is unacceptable because it would put cancer surgeons like me out of business. Trust me, there would still be plenty of surgical business. The real reason that chemo rarely plays a role in primary tumor treatment is based on facts and physiology. The majority of primary tumors, and even many metastases, are simply too large to be completely killed off by circulating chemo drugs. Blood flow within larger malignant growths frequently does not allow for chemo drugs to accumulate to high enough concentrations to kill all of the cancer cells. Thus, chemo frequently *shrinks* primary tumors or large mets, but it rarely completely destroys all of the cancer cells composing a primary tumor or large met. (Chemo *can* serve as primary treatment for a small number of primary tumor types, such as anal cancer, especially when combined with radiation treatment; however, these are far and away the minority of malignancies.) To achieve chemo drug levels within a primary tumor or large met that are high enough to kill every cancer cell, the toxicity of the chemo would be intolerable to the patient's normal tissues. Thus, chemo is only rarely used (and often in conjunction with radiation therapy) in an attempt to non-surgically cure a primary tumor or large metastasis.

CHEMOTHERAPY FOR DISTANT METASTATIC DISEASE VERSUS REGIONAL LYMPH NODE SPREAD

While you've just learned that chemo will likely be recommended if you have gross distant and/or microscopic regional lymphatic metastatic disease, there is a significant difference between these two "chemo indications" in terms of your prognosis (chance of survival and cure). *Many types of cancer that have spread to regional lymph nodes are still curable (with chemo playing a critical role) as long as there is no identified distant spread (M0).* Sadly, the reverse is not true: *If distant mets are found (M1), your chance of ultimately surviving your cancer drops precipitously regardless of your regional lymph node status.* However, even if the likelihood of cure is low (or in some cases, nonexistent), you will likely still be offered chemotherapy in an attempt to *prolong* your life. This is a tricky area, and if you are in this unfortunate position, you must carefully discuss with your oncologist and your family the true "pluses and minuses" of receiving chemo to potentially extend your life. At the heart of the matter is an appreciation that the potential for "prolonged life" is often measured in months and may or may not be worth the likely side effects associated with receiving the chemo. Is an additional two months with your family worth constant, severe nausea throughout that extra time? For some of you the answer is yes; for others, no. *These are very personal choices that should not be left to your oncologist but, rather, should be decided by you and your loved ones.* And do not forget: If you choose to start chemo in hopes of adding some quality time to your life and it turns out that the chemo makes you miserable, you can choose to stop receiving the chemo and enjoy your remaining time without any more chemo side effects (they usually wear off quickly). Because you have ultimate control to change your mind at any time, if you are a "terminal cancer patient," choosing to at least start chemo in the hope that you will gain additional, valuable, quality time with family and friends may well be a reasonable option.

Now, *a very lucky few who are found to have positive distant metastases may still have a chance at being cured.* Such curative treatment for M1 disease frequently depends on surgical removal of all gross metastatic disease (therefore, the total number and location of all distant mets is critical in identifying the handful of patients with a shot at cure). (The surgeon who is most qualified to remove your metastatic cancer may not be the surgeon who resected your primary tumor, depending on the location of your cancer spread.) Even if surgery removes all of your known distant mets, you'll still almost certainly receive additional chemotherapy once you've recovered from your operation. Why? Clearly your cancer metastasizes, and it is foolish to believe that the only metastases in your body were the ones large enough to be seen and then removed by your surgeon. *You must assume that additional small clusters of cancer cells remain in distant sites*, and left untreated, these will blossom into larger mets, making your survival very unlikely.

How Do You Decide Whether or Not to Accept Chemo Treatment?

As I've said about so many aspects of your cancer ownership, the decision to accept your oncologist's recommendation to receive chemotherapy should be *your decision*, not your oncologist's decision. As strongly as your doctor or doctors push chemo, theirs is still a professional *recommendation*. Only you can make the decision, as it is your cancer. Now much of the time, the decision to follow their recommendation is one you should obviously accept. If without chemo the risk of cancer recurrence is high, and if that risk is significantly reduced with chemotherapy, you should take the chemo. But even here, the terms "high" and "significantly reduced" are uncomfortably vague and flexible. While a 95 percent risk of cancer recurrence is clearly "high," is an 8 percentage-point reduction (to an 87 percent risk of cancer recurrence) a "significant reduction" worthy of the potential side effects and risks associated with chemo administration? Is a 12 percent risk of cancer recurrence "low," and if so, would you risk the toxicity if the addition of chemo reduced that risk to 6 percent (a 50 percent risk reduction)? *Only you (with input from your loved ones and oncologist) can determine for you* the definition of a "high risk" of cancer recurrence if you decline chemotherapy and the definition of a "significant reduction" in cancer recurrence risk if you accept chemo treatment. And these two definitions must be considered together, along

The decision to accept your oncologist's recommendation to receive chemotherapy should be your decision, not your oncologist's. with the toxicity profile (potential side effects and risks) of the proposed chemotherapy regimen. These considerations may be further complicated if more than one chemo regimen option is available for your type and stage of cancer, as each regimen will have its own toxicity profile. Thus, sometimes defining and weighing the potential benefits and risks of chemo may feel a bit like shooting at the proverbial moving target. Still, as the owner of the cancer, your goal remains despite all of these challenges: to first define what the risk of cancer recurrence with and without chemotherapy means to you; and then, if you have decided to follow the chemo recommendation, to select (if more than one chemo regimen is offered) the chemo regimen with the toxicity profile that seems to you the least unpleasant and/or least likely to occur.

Keep two important things in mind when making these decisions (as if you didn't have enough to consider already):

1. As I shared with you previously, while I discourage it in all but the most extreme cases, *you can always stop chemo treatment whenever you wish*, and your side effects will likely rapidly disappear; but

2. More important, if your cancer recurs, it is likely to kill you.

So, are you the kind of person who will be more comfortable with yourself if you decide not to follow the recommendation to receive chemo and then your cancer recurs, given that it might have recurred even if you *had* accepted chemotherapy? Or are you the kind of person who will be more comfortable if you take the chemo and your cancer does not recur, but you'll never know if the chemo (which may have made you miserable during treatment) had anything to do with your survival. Far and away, most of you (of us all) are the second kind of people (the ones who say yes to chemo), but it is your choice.

SELECTING YOUR CHEMO REGIMEN WHEN MORE THAN ONE IS OFFERED

Often more than one chemo regimen (combination of chemotherapy drugs) is available to treat your type and stage of cancer. There are literally hundreds of chemotherapy agents and thousands of regimens, resulting in a chemotherapy world that is simply overwhelming, even for many oncologists. So if more than one chemo approach is available to treat your type and stage of cancer, how do you partner with your oncologist to pick the right regimen for you? Many times your doctor will recommend one chemo regimen over the others based on his or her own professional experience with patients who own your type and stage of cancer. If you have selected the right oncologist for you, her/his recommendation should carry significant weight as you make your decision. But remember that knowledge is power, so doing a little research on your own will help you make this important treatment decision.

You know that chemo kills cancer cells, and you also know that chemo may be toxic to some normal tissues, resulting in the risk of side effects and even serious complications. When comparing chemo regimens, first recognize that they're all acceptable options because *no one regimen has demonstrated a greater likelihood of cure* (or else this would be the *only* option). So you must perform an analysis comparing the potential side effects and health risks of the differing available chemo regimens. In making such toxicity-profile comparisons, there are a couple of factors to consider. First, you must understand the *incidence* of the side effects and complications associated with a specific treatment regimen. Incidence really means how many treated patients experience this undesired outcome, and it's usually expressed as a percentage. Thus, a 2 percent incidence of severe nausea means that two out of every one hundred patients receiving the regimen developed severe nausea (the definition of "severe" may be a bit vague, but it is still clearly not something you would wish on your daughter's mohawk-wearing boyfriend). Next, you must appreciate the side effects and complications *themselves*. Side effects are things like nausea, hair loss, weight loss, fatigue (tiredness). While these may be hard to endure, they are temporary, and while they may be uncomfortable or even miserable, they rarely truly threaten your long-term health or life. *Complications*, on the other hand, may be more serious, may impact your health long-term, and very rarely may even threaten your life. Liver failure, kidney failure, and a significant reduction in your infection-fighting capability are examples of complications. So again, you must weigh apples and oranges. Which is worse: a 15 percent incidence of severe headache and a 2 percent risk of temporary kidney failure, or a 12 percent incidence of nausea, 2 percent incidence of hair loss, and 0.5 percent risk of permanent nerve damage in the hands and feet? *How the hell does anyone choose between these apples and oranges* (even an oncologist)? A lot of it is simply a gut call based on your oncologist's impression of how their previous patients have tolerated the different treatments. Depending on their age and experience and your type and stage of cancer, your oncologist's recommendations may be based only on what regimens their oncologist teachers prescribed; the oncologist may rarely or even never have used some of the recommended chemo regimens. Listen, there are thirty "headache pills" lining the shelves of your local pharmacy. Do you own one of every bottle? After all, they're all approved by the FDA, and all supposedly work to reduce your headache. No. You like aspirin. Or Tylenol. Or Motrin. Or one or two others. And you stick with those one or two because you know through your experience that they work, so why change? It's the same for chemo regimens. But you should not count solely on your oncologist's experience. You should weigh that experience heavily, but add your own knowledge to the decision pool.

But you may ask, how in the hell are you going to find and then understand all of this complex information, let alone use this information to make an informed decision? Take a breath. You can do this—and your family can help. The best way to learn and understand the basic chemo information and then weigh what you have learned is through reading (on credible Internet sites and in credible cancer books) and through multiple detailed (even if repetitive) discussions with your oncologist. Be prepared to hear a great deal of often confusing information. I strongly suggest that you *have a friend or loved one with you during these discussions with your oncologist,* and that the friend or loved one take notes. Such an approach will allow you to have a written record for later review. And don't be afraid to ask questions. Lots of questions. Even repeatedly. Keep asking them until you understand what you need to understand to make the best decision for you. And even then, keep in mind it's a guessing game, as some people have no side effects when receiving highly toxic chemo drugs while others are extremely sensitive and suffer miserable side effects from usually mild chemo agents. You won't know how your body will react, but you can make your decision based heavily on your oncologist's experience and guidance as well as on what you've learned. And remember that even side effects that are seemingly intolerable will be over within a relatively short time (though it may not seem "short" to you), but you'll never get over dying from your cancer should you abandon treatment.

And also remember, much of the complexity and your limited experience regarding the selection of your chemo regimen are mitigated by seeking a recommendation through doctors who believe and participate in a Tumor Board (as discussed previously in the chapter on doctor and medical center selection). The Tumor Board will hash out the different chemo options based on the personal preferences and experiences of multiple participating cancer doctors, offering you a consensus treatment recommendation. Even then, you can select another accepted, offered treatment. *You own it,* so the decision is yours.

Let's Talk "Cure"

Now that we've gotten deep into the varying aspects of cancer treatment, let's talk cure. Cure. Your goal. Your physicians' goal. What does "cure" mean, exactly? For most, cure means no longer having any cancer cells living within your body. Therefore, your cancer cannot kill you now and cannot return ever. Sounds good. Sounds like a winner.

But physicians don't routinely talk about cure. Rather, we talk of "survival," usually five-year survival. By talking about survival rather than cure, we're hedging our bets. How? Well, if we believe we've removed all of your cancer, but three years later your cancer "returns," you may *survive* five years, but in years four and five you'll have cancer that may kill you in year six or seven. Thus "survival" does not equal "cure." *The physicians' real term for "cure" is "disease-free survival" (or "cancer-free survival").* In the last example, the patient survived five years but had a three-year disease-free survival. Thus, when discussing your prognosis (future) with your doctors, you need to understand whether you are discussing "survival" or "disease-free survival."

When physicians speak of survival, we also speak of its evil twin: *recurrence*. Recurrence means a return of your cancer. For many of you (and I wish for all of you), the stage at which your cancer is initially diagnosed means there is a likelihood of curing you. (For those of you who were initially diagnosed with an advanced-stage cancer for which cure is either highly unlikely or impossible, we'll discuss treatment considerations later in this chapter.) To achieve that cure, you may undergo surgery, radiation therapy, and/or chemotherapy. By the time your treatment is completed, you and your doctors will, hopefully, believe that you've been cured, that there are no living cancer cells left within your body. But *for many cancer patients, the belief that they are "cured" is, sadly, temporary.*

Small groups of cancer cells may survive your "curative" treatment, hiding within your liver, lungs, and/or elsewhere. Too small to have been detected on your original imaging studies or during your surgery, these clusters of viable (living, growing) cancer cells survived the bombardment of radiation and the toxicity of your chemotherapy treatment. So they'll continue to multiply, the clusters growing. They may be metastases, or they may have survived at the site of your primary tumor (or, rarely, both). They may even send off more malignant cells through your bloodstream to form additional metastases.

It is this risk of the unknown, of viable cancer cells still surviving, hiding out after you have undergone curative treatment, that drives our aggressive "patient follow-up" strategies. We are searching, ever vigilant for evidence of a recurrence, looking for the return of your disease as surviving cancer cells reach numbers and size that allow for their identification on your scheduled follow-up CAT scan or chest X-ray, or their detection as an elevated "biomarker" (a protein released by certain types of cancers) on your scheduled follow-up blood tests. It is not within the purview of this book to dive into the details of follow-up strategies. Rather, I just want you to understand a few key things:

- Even if the attempt at curative treatment appears to have succeeded, your doctors will be following up with you regularly per recognized, accepted follow-up protocols, searching for evidence of cancer recurrence (failure to cure).

- Each type (and to a lesser extent, stage) of cancer has its own follow-up strategy.

- Depending on your cancer and treatment, follow-up may be performed by your oncologist and/or surgeon (radiation therapy follow-up is rarely indicated).

- Cancer recurrences don't occur linearly; that is, your chance of recurrence is not the same at year one, year two, year three, and year four following treatment. For most cancers, the majority of recurrences occur within two years following initial treatment, with virtually all recurrences occurring within five years following initial treatment. In such cases, I recommend a big dinner out (with champagne) for you, your spouse, and your kids on your second-year anniversary, and a blow-out block party for everyone you know on your fifth anniversary (don't spend all your money, as now you're gonna live for a long, long time). However, check with your oncologist to understand the timing of recurrences for your specific type and stage of cancer. Sadly, for a few types of cancer (including some common types), you can't have a party at two or even five years.

I share all of this stuff about recurrence not to scare you, but to help you understand your physicians when they recommend treatment options and follow-up strategies to you. You must decide which path to take, but you need to understand that they'll be talking about "recurrence rates" as well as "survival rates" and "disease-free survival rates." I say that disease-free survival and recurrence are simply "bookends," opposites of each other. If a treatment offers a "70 percent five-year disease free survival rate," it also means that 30 percent of those receiving the treatment suffered a recurrence of their malignancy within five years of that treatment (and it doesn't indicate what percentage of those 30 percent who recur are alive at five years, something you may wish to ask). Own your cancer and ask for clarity from your doctors in this all-important discussion. Make 100 percent certain that you understand exactly what each outcome with which you are presented truly means. *Write it down (in your own words) while your doctors present the outcomes, and then ask your doctors to read and verify that what you've written down is correct.*

What About Refusing All Treatment?

No doubt about it, refusing potentially cancer-curing treatment is the ultimate expression of cancer ownership. And shooting your pickup truck multiple times with your assault rifle because the battery's dead is the ultimate expression of truck ownership (not to mention your Second Amendment right) . . . but in my opinion, doing either also likely means you're an idiot.

Yes, cancer treatment can be miserable, especially recovering from surgery and enduring chemo. And yes, radiation and chemo treatments can last for months and months and months. And yes, you might not be able to work for a long time. Or golf. Or take a trip to Europe. Or make love to your spouse. And it's true, you may need to actually ask for help from others. *And it may not work, and you may still end up dying from your cancer.*

A couple of points here. First, put away your assault rifle, buy a new battery for your truck, and stop acting like a jackass. You've been presented with both the potential negatives (risk of side effects and complications) and the potential positive (the likelihood that you will be cured). You know that if you find the risks and toxicity too great for the potential survival benefit, you can always refuse any further treatment (other than once you're asleep for surgery). And you certainly know all of the reasons to go for it: your spouse, your kids, your parents, your dog, your friends, golfing, fishing, traveling . . . hell, even work. Put bluntly: I have yet to hear a reasonable explanation for refusing to at least *begin* undergoing a standard cancer treatment plan that provides a patient with a reasonable chance of cure. Trust me, I am *not* a "life is always worth living, no matter what" kind of guy. I worked the phones in a Suicide and Crisis Center when I was in college, and the first thing they taught us in our long hours of training was that some people who call you from the bridge at two in the morning, who just want to hear one last voice before they jump, do *not* actually have "a reason to live." After talking with them for an hour, searching for the tiniest glimmer of light to draw them out of the darkness, any iota of meaning or value in their day-to-day existence that is "worth living for," you come to realize that for them, simply saying good-bye, hanging up the phone, and jumping may be an entirely reasonable plan. *But that's not you.* The day before you were diagnosed with your cancer, you weren't calling me from a bridge. You were driving your kid to soccer, commiserating with your spouse over the bills, laughing with your pals, whatever. So *start the treatment and get back to it*. Own your cancer . . . it's the best way to own your life.

But what if you and your doctors agree that the likelihood of cure with the proposed "best treatment plan" is very low and the risks and toxicity of the treatment regimen are very high. What then? Again I remind you: *Other than when you go to sleep for surgery, you control when and if you continue to receive all nonsurgical therapy*. If indeed the side effects are horrific, so horrific that they outweigh the small likelihood of success, stop the treatment. You'll feel better by Thursday, and you can know that you gave it your best. That said, I do understand that if you suffer an irreversible treatment complication (such as a surgical complication or a chemo-related infection), it may further reduce your quality of life during your limited remaining time. Fortunately, such permanent complications are uncommon—but you still have to consider them, because if it happens to you, it doesn't matter how "uncommon" a complication is. In these situations you must truly own your cancer and make the decision for yourself. You must decide whether for you, and *no one knows you better than you*, it is right to risk treatment complications and toxicity for a very low chance of gaining any more time, or to accept that you will ultimately die from your cancer and doing with your remaining time as you see fit (which may be deciding not to spend some of that precious time sitting in the chemotherapy bay or in the radiation treatment room or puking into the toilet).

Again, this is truly your choice—no one knows you better than you know you—but you absolutely should seek the counsel, input, advice, and thoughts of others. Particularly your spouse and your family. And perhaps a close friend or two, and maybe your minister, priest, rabbi, or whomever. And then share your thoughts with your doctor. Good cancer doctors have cared for patients who have declined treatment, and we often both understand and support such a decision. Rest assured, we don't abandon you. We shift our focus of care to palliation if necessary, hospice if appropriate, and support for you and your family through to the end.

Sometimes it truly is better to say "no thank you" to the treatment offer and hop on a plane to Hawaii with your spouse and kids.

Recurrent Cancer

Far and away *the most common cause of cancer death is the result of recurrent disease.* As I've said before, "recurrent" cancer is a poor term, as it suggests a new cancer that develops after your original cancer has been cured. In reality, cancer recurrence simply represents malignant cells that survived your initial treatment and continued to multiply, eventually growing to a size and/or numbers that became detectable on imaging studies, blood tests (less commonly), and/or based on new complaints (such as pain) or physical findings (such as yellowing called jaundice). *Cancer recurrence at a distant metastatic site is the most frequent cause of cancer-related deaths.*

Your first shot at curing your cancer is far and away your best shot at curing your cancer.

However, cancer can also recur locally (at the site of the original primary tumor), within the region (arising from cancer that survived within lymph nodes or other regional tissues not removed during surgery), or in any combination of local-regional-distant.

A single statement cannot overemphasize why it is so critical to initially select the right doctors, undergo the correct initial surgical procedure, and receive the most appropriately aggressive radiation and chemotherapy: *Your first shot at curing your cancer is far and away your best shot at curing your cancer.*

Should your cancer recur, your chance of survival drops precipitously, even with aggressive treatment. Only a small group of recurrent cancer patients are even eligible for a second attempt at curative treatment. For the majority of cancers, attempted cure almost always heavily depends on the ability to remove all gross disease surgically, and there are very strict criteria regarding the number and/or size of mets that qualify you for such an attempt. Even those few folks who are deemed eligible for another attempt at cure for the majority of cancers are often found at surgery to have much more extensive metastatic disease than identified by imaging studies prior to surgery, and the surgery is abandoned.

In our earlier discussion about refusal of treatment, where I strongly encouraged you to seriously consider treatment even if the likelihood of cure was low, we were talking about initial (first-time) treatment. When faced with recurrent cancer, which has already successfully fought against your initial attempt to kill it, the discussion is a bit different. The cancer has history on its side. That doesn't mean I am encouraging those of you who develop recurrent cancer to simply throw in the towel on day one. You should immediately be evaluated for *eligibility* for an attempted cure of your recurrent disease, which usually involves imaging studies to identify metastases in all the places that are common targets for your specific cancer type. Such an evaluation is safe and painless and generates a binary result: You are either ineligible for attempted cure (the overwhelming majority of patients), or you are in the small population who still appear eligible for attempted cure. If you're among the latter, remember that only a fraction of eligible patients are ultimately cured ("eligible" does not equal "curable"). Here again, you must decide whether or not to undergo another operation and additional chemotherapy (which may be more toxic than your initial chemo, given the need to step up the aggressiveness of your attack) and, potentially, additional radiation. Speak with your loved ones and others throughout your support network. Read from *credible* sources about the treatment of your type of cancer when it recurs. Speak openly and honestly with all of the physicians who would be involved in this second treatment program (surgeon, oncologist, and, if included, rad onc). And then decide. There is no generally acknowledged "right choice" here. There is only a right choice *for you*. And only you can make that right choice.

If you are in the much larger group of folks with recurrent cancer who are ineligible for a second attempt at cure, you also have a decision to make: additional treatment or no additional treatment. You may ask, if you're not curable, why would you undergo additional treatment? First of all, if the recurrence is causing you problems (pain, bleeding, obstruction, etc.), you may wish to consider "palliative treatment," which we'll discuss in the next section. But if your recurrent cancer is causing no problems, as is often the case when it is initially discovered (usually on imaging studies), why undergo more therapy? Because now you know that your cancer is going to be the cause of your death, and now we're talking about *time*. Sometimes additional treatment (almost always chemo, but sometimes radiation as well) can potentially offer you additional time, usually measured in months but sometimes measured in longer periods. That said, additional chemo (which may be more toxic than your initial failed chemo) carries the potential for side effects and complications that *may reduce your quality of life during some or all of that additional time*. Yep. Same challenge. You must weigh the potential benefit of added time to spend with those you love and doing things you love against how crappy more chemo may make you feel (which may limit how much time you are truly able to spend with the people and doing the activities you love). Again remember, you can always start chemo and if your quality of life tanks to the point that it's not worth the potential extra few months, *you can always choose to stop receiving treatment* and you'll feel better soon. *It is and must remain your choice.* And unlike that tiny group of people who terminate chemo during their *initial* attempt at cure (which causes everyone to shake their heads), deciding to terminate chemo when you are incurable will cause no reaction other than support for your having given it a try.

Palliative Treatment

To "palliate" something means "to lessen the severity without curing or removing." When we speak of palliative treatment, we are admitting that:

1. You are either refusing treatment attempting cure or have been evaluated as incurable (either due to advanced disease at initial diagnosis or recurrent cancer), and

2. Local, regional, and/or distant disease is causing you problems (such as pain, bleeding, obstruction).

Not all symptoms and complaints that are produced by malignant disease can be palliated. Fortunately, some of the most miserable ones often can be. Pain (local or distant disease) can frequently be reduced with radiation therapy. Some "external" bleeding (blood in your urine or stool, for example) resulting from tumor growth can also be reduced and controlled with radiation; however, surgery may be required to end bleeding resulting from malignant disease. Obstruction (of the intestines, urine-carrying ureters, esophagus, etc.) most often requires surgery to palliate, although some nonsurgical **stents** (tubes that hold open whatever body structure a cancer is trying to block) and even radiation therapy may be able to provide acceptable palliation in a limited number of obstruction scenarios. If surgery is the only approach to palliating your symptoms, you will first need to have serious discussions with your surgeon *to determine whether you are healthy enough to undergo the palliative operation*. Know the real risks, given your current state of health. For some people, there is no alternative to palliative surgery other than death (a completely obstructed intestine, significant ongoing bleeding), and if that death will likely be painful, many of these people would rather die comfortably during or soon after the palliative operation than die painfully from their disease. Even for non–life threatening pain, some people would rather risk a surgical death than a short life with that pain. As for chemotherapy, it plays virtually no role in palliative therapy other than its occasional use to enhance the potency of certain palliative radiation treatments.

Continue to own your cancer so you can continue to own your life.

165

These decisions are still yours and yours alone. *Incurable patients, too, should own their cancers.* I hope that you, dear reader, never have to face our inability to help you get cured. But if you do face this outcome, as some of you will, continue to own your cancer so you can continue to own your life, and if your cancer is causing you unremitting pain or dangerous bleeding or another problem that cannot be controlled with medications, there is no harm in asking your physicians about palliative treatment options. And don't ask the oncologist about surgical palliation, because they're likely not to admit that they don't know; ask your surgeon about surgical palliation and your rad onc about radiation therapy palliation. Many of my patients have found comfort and peace in their final months or years as a result of palliative treatment. It allowed them to live out their remaining life on their terms.

Getting a Second Opinion

Why didn't I place this section on second opinions earlier in this chapter? Because I don't want you to think that a second opinion is of value only when you are taking your first shot at curing your cancer. Second opinions may be very helpful to any of you who now have a recurrent cancer, for those readers who are considering refusing treatment, and also for those of you who are wondering whether palliative treatment would help or even be possible. The usefulness of a second opinion is not limited to the potentially curable cancer owner selecting their initial treatment strategy. Okay. Now keep reading.

Even assuming that you've selected your doctors in a thoughtful way (as guided by this book), once you hear a treatment recommendation from your surgeon, radiation oncologist, and/ or medical oncologist, and once you've asked your questions and heard their answers, you still may feel unconvinced—or at least concerned—that some or all aspects of the recommended treatment may not be right for you. Don't discount such feelings. Instead, you should seek a second opinion, defined as *seeking a treatment recommendation from a different physician*.

I recognize that obtaining a second opinion may be very difficult for many of you. After all, you don't want to "hurt your doctor's feelings" or "make your doctor angry." Remember, *it's all about you, baby*. And think about this: If the second opinion physician agrees with your doctor, then when you return to your doctor for treatment, your doctor feels pretty damn good about himself/herself. And if the second opinion disagrees with your doctor's recommendation, and you are more comfortable with the alternate treatment approach, then you'll switch physicians and receive the treatment that you feel is the right one for you. It's a win-win situation—most importantly, for you! And take it from a surgeon who knows: If you return to me because the second opinion is in agreement with my recommendation, I am not hurt or angry . . . *I am proud of you for owning your cancer and seeking input* (plus, I'm clearly brilliant).

There are a few important guidelines when seeking a second opinion regarding your surgical, radiation, and/or chemotherapeutic treatment recommendations:

- You must seek a second opinion from someone at least as experienced and interested in your type of cancer as your doctor.

- The doctor providing you a second opinion *cannot be a partner or direct colleague of your doctor*. Such a relationship often inhibits the second-opinion physician from disagreeing with your doctor (his colleague and, perhaps, friend). Go to a physician with no professional or personal relationship with your doctor. (Ask! Verify!)

- Don't be afraid to tell the second-opinion doctor who your physician is and what her/his recommended treatment is. With a few exceptions, physicians are all professionals and do not bad-mouth one another to patients, nor do we "steal" each other's patients. All that said, *consider sharing your doctor's recommendation only after hearing the recommendation of the second-opinion physician.* This avoids your doctor's recommendation having any impact (favorable or unfavorable; intentional or subconscious) on the second-opinion doctor.

- *Make certain that you understand if and how your medical insurance covers second opinions.* Many insurance plans do not cover any part of a payment for a second opinion. If your insurer covers little or nothing, then you have to decide whether your concern over your doctor's recommendation is worth the out-of-pocket cost for that second opinion (and you should feel very comfortable calling the second opinion office and asking the cost for a second-opinion visit). Here's my take: (1) you own your cancer, (2) the wrong choice may have dramatic negative consequences on your survival and quality of life, and (3) you can skip

McDonald's for the next ten years to pay for your second opinion, but you have to select the right treatment in order to be alive in ten years to finally eat another Big Mac. What the hell am I saying here? *If you are not comfortable with a treatment recommendation from any of your doctors, find the money and get the second opinion.* Even if the second opinion agrees with the original recommendation and you return to be treated by your doctor (a common outcome), *you will not have wasted your money.* After all, isn't "peace of mind" worth something when it comes to decisions about your survival?

- Finally, move the process along rapidly. Not only do you want (and need) to get your treatment started, it does annoy some physicians when their patient delays treatment for any length of time (an annoyance based on a concern that valuable time is being wasted). Thus, get that second opinion by the end of next week, okay? Explain to the nurse or receptionist on the phone that you are seeking a second opinion because you are scheduled to begin your cancer treatment in two weeks (or whenever you really are to begin treatment). Once you have an appointment scheduled, what really helps is providing ahead of time (at best) or bringing with you (at worst) copies of all of your medical records pertaining to your cancer, copies of imaging study (X-ray) reports, the actual imaging studies themselves (hospitals will put them all on a CD for you), and copies of all pathology reports (from any biopsies, surgery, etc.).

Remember, *all this medical information is legally yours and available with your signature.* That said, hospitals don't exist solely to serve you, so request these documents and X-rays as soon as you can, even if it means repeatedly pestering the staff in the medical records and radiology departments. They'll get over it. The squeaky wheel gets the grease. *It's all about you, baby.*

As I said at the start of this section, you may also wish to consider obtaining a second opinion if your doctors tell you there is no treatment option for you (you are "incurable"), if your cancer has recurred, or if you are interested in palliative therapy (either because you've been told that no palliative treatment is available or you wish to hear another option regarding what you've been offered). These three scenarios represent much more desperate situations than initial cancer treatment, and it never hurts to hear a second expert's perspective on your difficult situation.

All your medical information is legally yours and available with your signature.

Clinical Trials

In all of my experiences partnering with and guiding people through the maze that is cancer, perhaps no area has engendered so much confusion and such a challenge (both for patients and doctors) as clinical trials.

First of all, *what the hell is a clinical trial?* Whenever a pharmaceutical company develops a new chemotherapy drug, that company is required by the US Food and Drug Administration (FDA) to demonstrate that the new agent meets with agreed upon definitions of safety and effectiveness. For this discussion, we will focus on chemotherapeutic drugs (new radiation technology and surgical instrumentation must also prove safe and effective, but clinical trials of radiation and surgical equipment innovations are much less common). Now, new chemo drugs are first designed in laboratories using computer models, studies using cells, studies using animals, and other processes not involving human beings. But after closely reviewing these early (and very costly) research and development activities, at some time the company has to fish or cut bait. And by fish, I mean give the new chemo drug to some humans. Thus, "human subjects trials" are performed and are generically referred to as "clinical trials." There are several sequential clinical trial phases that must be performed for a drug manufacturer to ultimately get the thumbs-up from the FDA for commercial sale of the product to hospitals, clinics, and your doctor.

In **Phase I trials** (usually the earliest phase, although even earlier developmental Phase 0 trials are being introduced), a new chemo drug is tested in humans for the first time. Very few patients (often as few as twenty, and rarely greater than one hundred patients), who are called **subjects** in clinical trial lingo, are enrolled in a Phase I trial. These subjects are given different (increasing) doses of the new drug while the side effects (toxicity) of the differing drug doses are evaluated. A major goal of a Phase I clinical trial is to determine the highest dose of the new drug associated with an acceptable level of toxicity (side-effects).

There are other Phase I trial goals, such as understanding how the drug is absorbed by different body tissues, but the primary goal is to appreciate the toxicity of differing drug dosages. Thus, given that the effectiveness of the drug in fighting cancer in humans is unproven, and even the appropriate drug dose is unknown, *for most subjects, the likelihood of realizing any meaningful benefit in treating their cancer through participation in a Phase I clinical trial is very low.* (After reading that last sentence, Phase I clinical trial physicians, backed by the multinational pharmaceutical companies, are placing a large bounty on my head . . .). In my experience, two types of cancer owners participate in Phase I clinical trials. First are people with cancer who participate out of a true desire to help future cancer patients. For a new drug to prove truly beneficial in treating cancer, it must successfully complete Phase I evaluation and then progress through subsequent clinical trial phases. Thus, these altruistic cancer owners seek to achieve one selfless goal through Phase I trial participation: helping move the new treatment through the required process in the hope that the drug will prove beneficial to future sufferers of their same type of cancer. Other individuals I have seen participate in Phase I clinical trials are patients with clearly advanced or terminal malignancies who are unwilling to simply "throw in the towel." For these unfortunate folks, Phase I clinical trial participation offers the only hope of additional time with loved ones, albeit a slim hope. All the preceding notwithstanding, there are cases in which some Phase I clinical trial subjects have achieved remarkable results, in the form of significant quality time added to their lives. In the end, the decision of whether or not to participate in this, the earliest phase of new treatment development, is very, very personal.

Phase II clinical trials enroll more subjects than Phase I, but the number of participants remains small (again, typically fewer than one hundred). Phase II clinical trials continue the work of Phase I trials, further delineating the toxicity profile of the higher new drug doses while for the first time also evaluating potential new drug effectiveness. As with Phase I participation, enrolling in a Phase II Clinical Trial has a limited likelihood of personally benefitting you (although in a Phase II clinical trial, you'll certainly receive higher doses of the new drug than did many Phase I subjects). But again, your participation may allow the evaluation process to continue and, hopefully, prove the drug valuable to others suffering from your cancer in the future, and if you are suffering from advanced or terminal disease, enrollment in a Phase II trial may be the only option that provides you with the hope you are seeking.

For most, the likelihood of realizing any meaningful benefit in treating their cancer through participation in a Phase I clinical trial is very low.

If you are the type of individual who is willing to participate in a clinical trial that will likely not benefit you directly (and may even result in unpleasant side effects) but will be important in determining whether the drug may benefit other cancer owners in the future, then consider enrolling in a Phase I or a Phase II clinical trial—and from those of us who care for cancer patients, and from future cancer patients—*thank you* and *God bless you.* No kidding, no sarcasm. It is a true gift that you are giving to thousands of people you'll never know. And if you are someone suffering from advanced or terminal cancer for which there are few or no treatments being offered, and if you are still not ready to abandon all attempts to treat your disease (which is your right!), then enrollment in a Phase I or Phase II clinical trial may be a reasonable decision, and I truly hope that you are in that group who does benefit from participation. So now on to Phase III trials . . .

One very important thing to understand about participation in clinical trials: The new drug being studied is not administered alone. The new drug is given to you *along with the standard (proven and approved) treatment* for your type and stage of cancer. Thus, *you will not receive a lesser treatment than you would if you chose not to participate in a clinical trial.* This is because in the United States, clinical trials cannot include a group of participants who receive anything less than the "Standard of Care." And it is extremely uncommon for a new drug to reduce the effectiveness of the standard treatment. If you have advanced cancer for which no standard treatment is offered, you may receive only the investigational drug, but this is not commonly the case, particularly in later phase trials.

It is through participation in a Phase III clinical trial that you as an individual are most likely to directly benefit from a treatment that will otherwise not be available in time to help you.

If the results of the Phase I and subsequent Phase II clinical trials are deemed favorable by the FDA, a **Phase III clinical trial** enrolling hundreds and hundreds of patients at many sites will likely follow. *It is through participation in a Phase III clinical trial that you as an individual are most likely to directly benefit from a drug that will otherwise not be available to you in time for your treatment.* In this final trial phase, the new cancer drug is administered at the dosage selected based on the results of the previous two trial phases. Again, the new drug is not administered alone. So don't be afraid that you'll get a lesser treatment than you would have received had you chosen not to participate. If you are randomly assigned to the group of patients who are to receive the new cancer drug, *you will receive the new drug in addition to the standard therapy for your type and stage cancer.* I'll clarify this, because it is the "safety net" required in our great country that is not required in some other countries. For example, a Phase III clinical trial may randomly assign subjects to one of two groups: One group to receive the standard treatment plus the new drug being evaluated; the second group to receive the identical standard treatment plus a placebo (a fake drug that does nothing). Why the trickery? The placebo is added so that no participant has any clue whether they're receiving the new drug or the fake (the placebo, which often looks similar to the new drug being evaluated). This is because we know that subjects who *believe* they are receiving a new cancer drug even when actually receiving a placebo often experience side effects (negative outcomes) and even an improved quality of life (a positive outcome). Thus, placebos are included in many Phase III clinical trials *to help determine the real negatives and positives associated with taking the new drug.* As a result, such **blinded** (no subject knows what they are receiving) **double-arm** (two treatment groups) studies allow the clinical trial to meet its goal of determining whether receiving the standard treatment plus the new cancer drug results in a better outcome (such as fewer cancer recurrences in the first years following treatment) than the standard treatment alone.

So what benefit might you receive, and what are the risks associated with participation in a Phase III clinical trial? Most commonly, Phase III cancer trials are trying to prove that the new cancer drug (1) increases survival and/or (2) increases the time before cancer recurs (which obviously is worse than increased survival) relative to accepted standard treatment. A few Phase III cancer trials evaluate a new drug's ability to reduce the toxicity of the standard treatment or some other nonsurvival or nonrecurrence outcome, but for the most part, these new drugs are aimed at either increasing overall survival (cure) or increasing the time a patient survives following treatment before his or her cancer recurs (disease-free survival). You'll need to ask the physician presenting the Phase III clinical trial what outcome or outcomes (survival, disease-free survival, reduced toxicity, etc.) are the projected benefits of the new drug. Then ask about the *magnitude* of the potential beneficial effect (for example, does the previous Phase I and Phase II work suggest that increased disease-free survival is on the order of weeks, months, or years?). Often the presenting physician cannot provide even relatively concrete answers to these "potential benefit" questions simply because no one knows. But they may be able to share an educated guess related to the success of drugs chemically similar to the new cancer agent being studied. As to the potential risks, that information comes directly from the Phase I and, especially, Phase II clinical trial results, as these two early phases are primarily focused on drug toxicity, whereas Phase III is focused on effectiveness for a dosage with a toxicity profile known from the previous trial phases. Also keep in mind, even after you are enrolled and even participating (receiving treatment) in a clinical trial, *you can decide at any time that you no longer wish to participate without offering any reason for your withdrawal.* Furthermore, no physician or medical facility can deny you further standard treatment or "retaliate" in any way because you have withdrawn from a clinical trial.

No physician or medical facility can deny you further standard treatment or "retaliate" in any way because you have withdrawn from a clinical trial.

That's right—pull out anytime, no questions asked, and continue to be cared for as if you had never enrolled.

So, just as you've already heard me say over and over again in this book, you will need to weigh the potential benefits of enrolling in a Phase III clinical trial with the potential risks of participation. If the standard treatment has outcomes that you feel are acceptably favorable, and if the new cancer drug has a concerning toxicity profile, you may want to pass. On the other hand, if the standard treatment results do not sound very encouraging, you may want to enroll regardless of the toxicity profile. This will likely be your only opportunity to receive the new drug, as it is often years before an approved new drug hits the market following completion of a Phase III clinical trial.

Certainly if you have recurrent cancer or "incurable" cancer, you may wish to consider participating in a Phase III clinical trial, as it may offer the best chance of cure (for patients with recurrent cancer) or the best chance of increased survival time (for patients with recurrent cancer and those with incurable cancer). But again, even if you have incurable cancer, you must weigh the potential benefits (survival that is usually measured in months) versus potential risks (side effects that may make you feel like crap) of clinical trial participation.

So who gets offered the opportunity to participate in a clinical trial? Well, there are hundreds of clinical trials evaluating new drugs to treat a variety of cancer types and stages. That said, there are far fewer trials for cancer types and stages for which the currently approved treatments are relatively successful and tolerable. And it makes sense—why spend millions on developing a new drug to treat a cancer that is already successfully treatable using an approved and available drug or combination of drugs? There is greater potential financial return in developing new drugs to treat cancers for which currently approved treatments have poor outcomes or for cancers with no real current treatment options. Same is true for "orphan cancers," cancers that occur in only a limited number of people annually. While I truly wish that there were enough money available for research into treatment development for all cancer types and stages, I cannot criticize the pharmaceutical companies. I understand not spending limited financial resources to replace highly successful, safe, well-tolerated drugs or to develop drugs that may benefit five hundred cancer owners at the expense of tens of thousands with another type of malignancy. Given that their resources are limited, I want pharmaceutical firms to spend that research and development money creating drugs to treat more common cancer types and stages for which current drugs have limited or no success. Thus it is more common to find clinical trials offered to evaluate new drugs in patients with very advanced stage disease and more difficult-to-cure cancers than for early-stage cancers and for malignancies for which we already have pretty good treatments. However, there is an occasional clinical trial even for these early-stage and treatable cancers as well.

So where to go to find out about what if any clinical trials might be available to you? Designated cancer centers and true academic medical centers have as a stated goal the advancement of patient care through research. They almost always have clinical research nurses or clinical coordinators whose primary job is to enroll cancer patients into regional or national clinical trials in which their doctors and hospitals are participating. Thus, if you are receiving care at such a facility and are interested in learning whether you qualify for a clinical trial, simply ask your physician to speak to the nurse or coordinator who oversees clinical trial patient enrollment. If you are at a community hospital that does not have such a coordinated clinical trial enrollment process, you can go online to ClinicalTrial.gov, where well over 130,000 clinical trials at sites across the world are presented. Remember, *your local oncologist may be able to participate in a regional or national clinical trial*, because he or she may be allowed to use the same new clinical trial drug and protocol (they have to be formally trained on the trial, which often is not hard). So you may not have to travel to Rochester, Minnesota, in the middle of February (done that—not good) to participate in a clinical trial sponsored by the Mayo Clinic. Your local doctor or a regional oncologist may be able to support your participation in that same Mayo Clinic study where you live.

As I said earlier, participation in clinical trials is a pathway for helping future cancer owners, especially enrollment in early-phase trials. And as with being an organ donor, this is a truly amazing gift that some cancer owners share with us all. But for those of you who have proven treatment options with *good outcomes*, clinical trials should be evaluated with some caution; there certainly are a few good reasons to consider participation, but make certain that those are clearly understood before signing on the dotted line. For those of you with questionable, poor, or no good treatment options, Phase III clinical trial participation should be seriously considered.

One final note: As I mentioned at the start of this section, some clinical trials do not evaluate new drugs, they evaluate new equipment or even techniques of treatment. In addition, some clinical trials do not evaluate any type of newly developed *treatment*. These clinical trials evaluate newly developed **diagnostic tests.** For example, today companies are developing technologies and tests to determine whether your cellular DNA includes genes that make it more likely you'll respond to certain chemotherapy drugs. Other companies are developing genetics tests that more clearly determine your risk of cancer recurrence, thus potentially guiding treatment recommendations and follow-up. These and other innovative diagnostic tests are also often evaluated via clinical trials. In these clinical trials, the risks to you are often minuscule or nonexistent (you may have to give a blood sample, or a sample of your tumor may need to be analyzed, and you may need to undergo additional follow-up imaging studies) and the potential benefits may be significant (in our examples, determining which chemo drugs may best kill your cancer cells or your true recurrence risk). The point here is that *non-therapeutic (non-treatment) diagnostic clinical trials are much more likely to be safe and simple and may actually help you and, at worst, may help future cancer patients more than help you.* Consider participating.

Finally, Don't Go to Mexico

When I was practicing in San Diego, a man in his sixties asked to see me as soon as possible. As I learned within the first few minutes of meeting the man and his wife, he had recently been diagnosed with metastatic rectal cancer and had already seen several oncologists, a couple of radiation oncologists, and a general surgeon. They had all told him the same thing, he explained as we sat in my office, tears running down his wife's cheeks: His stage rendered him incurable, and no one had anything to offer him "other than enrollment in a clinical trial." He viewed participation in a clinical trial as akin to being a "guinea pig" (a common feeling, I told him, and not entirely invalid) and an option that would offer him no meaningful shot at a cure (very likely an accurate assessment, I agreed). And he had no intention of dying. Not yet.

So he asked me to help cure him.

Having reviewed his imaging studies, pathology reports, and having completed my physical examination of the gentleman, I gently told him and his wife that I could not cure him and recommended that, given his understandable and reasonable refusal to consider clinical trial participation, he and his wife think about how they would like to share their remaining short time together, and that they familiarize themselves with the local hospice (via my introduction) to determine whether that service might be of benefit to them at some future time. Finally, we discussed the possible complications that could arise from his cancer and for which there might be palliative treatment. Then we softly discussed the likely manner in which he would die, when the time came.

And then the man and his wife graciously thanked me and left.

And then they went to Mexico.

Now, I didn't know at the conclusion of that first meeting that the man and his wife would be heading down to Mexico. If I had known, I might have thought little of it, given that we all traveled on occasion from San Diego to Mexico, with the border less than an hour away and the fresh lobster and beer awfully cheap. Plus, hadn't I just encouraged this couple to find ways to enjoy their remaining time together? A lot of people enjoy Mexico. So I would likely not have given it much thought, had I known that the man and his wife, upon leaving my office, were returning home to quickly pack their bags and head across the border.

I didn't know, and it didn't matter. Until I saw the man and his wife again about six weeks later. He was now prisoner-of-war thin ("cachectic"), his eyes deeply sunken in, his breathing shallow, his arms just skin and bone. But it wasn't his dramatic physical deterioration that startled me—after all, I had cared for many end-stage cancer patients, and the changes in his body were neither new to me nor unanticipated. I was startled by his total loss of spirit, and by the additional stress that showed in his wife's eyes and manner. And I knew these changes weren't solely, if even largely, because they now recognized the terminal course his disease was taking. They had known before. Even before they heard it from the third doctor or the sixth doctor.

I examined the man and then sat down across from the two of them. "What's happened since I saw you last?" I asked. They understood that my question was not about his progressive physical deterioration.

They had traveled to Mexico, they told me. He had read on the Internet about a miraculous cure for all types of terminal cancers, a novel treatment that "purged the blood and body of all cancer cells." The Internet site stated critically that the US FDA was "too focused on complicated, long-term clinical trials demonstrating effectiveness," so the treatment was "not yet available" in the States.

When I was nine years old, I went to overnight summer camp. There, I indulged in my passion for horses and horseback riding. You have to understand, a Jewish boy raised in the San Francisco Bay Area who loved caring for and riding horses was an anomaly. But at summer camp, nestled within the Santa Cruz Mountains, I was a member of a large community of boys and girls who loved horses just as I did. And I was good at it (at least as good as a nine-year-old who is around horses for four weeks a year can be). For three summers in a row, I returned to camp, counting the days during the school year until I could ditch my tennis shoes and pull on the boots that defined me as a true wrangler. By the time I attended camp as an eleven-year-old, I was a pretty good rider, and I had a general knack for horse care. Then the head wrangler, Trudy, made me an offer. She said that the camp owners were always open to having their better junior wrangler campers each care for one of the horses during the school year. For the owners, it meant one less horse who had to be reacquainted with the joys of carrying abusive children for six hours a day after nine months of freedom in the wild of the pasture. For the junior wrangler, it was a chance to have a horse of their own for nine whole months without having to come up with the cash to buy one. And so Trudy asked me if I wanted to care for Pogo for the nine months between that summer and the next summer. I could barely contain my excitement. That night, I immediately penned a letter to my parents that opened with, "Please, please, please don't say no . . ."

My parents knew as much about horses as they did about Norwegian ice fishing (no, they're neither Norwegian nor inclined to fish . . . and ice? We lived in California). I knew that. And I knew that the closest stable to our suburban home was a good twenty-minute drive up into the hills. And I knew that to properly care for Pogo, I'd have to see him every day after school and at least once every weekend. *I knew all of this*. And because even at eleven I thought too "scientifically" to simply ignore what I knew to be factual, my mind simply worked around the facts, developing a new reality and fooling my desiring mind into believing it was a rational plan. "I can bike to the stables every day after school," I pleaded when my parents came to visit mid-session. The bike trip would take me two hours each way, my mother pointed out. "It's uphill," my dad said. "Both ways." But I had convinced myself that I could do it, and that I could have Pogo for my own for nine whole months. *My own horse!*

My mind had taken all of my eleven years of experiences and, when driven by my unrealistic yet unshakable goal, forced itself to achieve my goal through the creation and acceptance of a "rational" strategy.

My patient was an intelligent man with a long life's worth of experiences. He had been told repeatedly, and no doubt appreciated deep inside, that he would soon die of his advanced rectal disease, that there was no cure for his cancer. So his mind simply forced him to accept the "rationality" of the only pathway he could identify that would allow him to reach his unrealistic yet unshakable goal, to be cured. And so he and his wife traveled to Mexico, where he repeatedly paid large sums of money (each payment in the tens of thousands of dollars), all taken from their nest egg, to the "clinician." And where he sat in a dirty room and watched his blood travel out of his frail arm through an intravenous line and into a box that was covered with lights and gauges and other technical-looking gadgets, and then back out of the box through the intravenous line and back into his other arm.

Of course the box through which his blood passed was just that—a box. Had you or I or any other competent individual without terminal cancer simply glanced for five seconds at the box, we would have laughed at the obvious hoax as we walked out of the room. But this competent man, my patient, had terminal cancer and a required outcome (cure), and so he saw a miracle. And he and his wife paid for it.

And when the "clinician" informed him following his initial three "treatments" that they were "clearly making progress," but that his cancer was "so aggressive that many additional treatments were needed," he and his wife excitedly *took out a second mortgage* on their California home and paid the additional $100,000-plus fee for the subsequent box purification treatments that would "save his life."

His last curative box purification treatment had been administered the same way as all of his previous dozen treatments only a few days before I saw him that second time. During his last weeks in Mexico, while they drained his savings account faster than they drained his blood, he and his wife finally understood the reality of their situation and the horrible impact of their last "rational" actions. Just as I, alone in the dark of my bunk those many, many summer nights ago, knew that I could never ride to and from the stables each day to care for my horse. Not even once. Come on . . . two hours . . . up hills? I was eleven. And I wasn't an idiot.

So the true sadness I saw on the man's face and the new stress so visible in his wife's eyes at that second, our final, visit was not solely because both had accepted the reality of his impending death. It was the realization that in the few short weeks since we had first met, their need to attain an unattainable outcome had cost them all of her future financial security, jeopardizing the well-being and quality of life for his wife once her beloved husband had died. Both were terrified not only for him because he was going to die soon, but for her, because she was going to struggle to live.

In all my years caring for all my cancer patients, this lesson was one of the saddest I learned, and one I swore not to forget. So I'll tell you what I have told virtually every patient with widely metastatic or locally recurrent terminal disease since that day: Consider enrolling in a clinical trial. Consider taking a trip with your wife to visit every major league ballpark in the National League. Consider sitting on the couch with your kids watching your favorite movies. Consider these and a thousand other things. Even consider visiting Mexico. *Just never open your checkbook, pull out your credit card, or withdraw cash because you've found a "cure."*

Needless to say, Pogo spent those nine months running around free in some pasture. I spent those nine months playing football with my friends after school. And counting the days until summer.

10

I Think I'll Just Drink
Wheat Grass Juice

Let's just get this out of the way right from the get-go: I am a proponent of Western medicine. And by "Western," I mean "modern," "scientific," "the best."

That doesn't mean that I believe in every Western approach recommended to every cancer patient. I know from my own practice that much of medical care delivered by physicians (including cancer care) is an art rather than a science. Even much of the science is unclear or controversial. At its core, Western medicine is an approach to care based on scientific evidence, a requirement for the objective demonstration of effectiveness, safety, and outcome. Western medicine ignores faith, hope, bias (at least these are the goals). Being 100 percent "Western" means that given the choice between chemotherapy for node positive breast cancer and spells cast by a witch doctor, I'll go for the chemo. Problem is, when it comes to "alternative medical treatments," it's not always as clear as chemo versus the witch doctor. Some alternative therapies claim to have objectively demonstrated their effectiveness and safety. And some truly have.

Alternative. The word itself implies something different than the standard. In our 24/7 Internet/Facebook/Twitter world, stories of lifesaving, side effect–free, miraculous "alternative" cancer therapies abound. If you search the Internet, you'll find websites that claim, "Read this information by someone who beat a stage 4 cancer by using the cancer-fighting strategies covered on this website." These reports are at such odds with what your doctor tells you about cancer that one of the biggest things you have to wrap your mind around is the obvious thought, "If the information in this report and the supplements recommended are so good, why isn't everyone using them?" It's a good question. Many alternative practitioners will tell you the answer is physician greed, and secondarily, that it takes a great deal of time for new ways to fight disease to be accepted. Yep, that's right. They hold that if we cancer doctors ever allow you, our patients, to realize that all it takes is a glass of wheat grass juice to cure your disease, we're screwed. How will we feed our children? No, we simply can't let you learn of the safe, simple, guaranteed cancer cures offered by "alternative therapies." Oh yeah . . . and the US Food and Drug Administration is in on it, too.

Come on. You're smarter than that!

Or are you? Because even the most intelligent, rational person can lose perspective when threatened with cancer. And it's understandable. Fear can powerfully influence rational thought. Fear of side effects. Fear of dying. Who wouldn't want a better "alternative"? One that promises no nausea or vomiting. One that promises you'll keep your hair. One that guarantees a cure. *It sounds too good to be true!*

It is.

The Four Rules

Here's the scoop. There are, in my experience, two broad categories of cancer treatments other than those offered by Western medicine: alternative therapies and supplemental therapies. I suggest my Four Rules to allow you to simply differentiate between *alternative* treatments (which I strongly oppose) and *supplemental* treatments (which I may not always endorse but I do not oppose):

1. The "therapy" is not recommended as a replacement for any or all of the treatments recommended by your cancer physicians;

2. The "therapy" does not reduce or in any way negatively impact the effectiveness (or have the potential to do so, according to your cancer physicians) of any or all of the treatments recommended by your cancer physicians;

3. The "therapy" does not delay your receiving any or all of the treatments recommended by your cancer physicians;

4. The "therapy" does not significantly drain your wallet.

The first three rules allow you to differentiate between "alternative" and "supplemental" cancer therapies. *If the therapy under consideration violates any one or more of these first three rules, it's an alternative therapy*, and regardless of the promises, the testimonials of the miraculously cured patients sharing their amazing, joyful stories on the website, *walk away*. If not one of the first three rules is violated, the therapy is likely supplemental. That doesn't mean you should jump at it; it only means that it is not unreasonable to proceed with caution—meaning a great deal of skepticism. (We'll talk a bit more about supplemental therapies later on in this chapter.)

And regardless of the other rules, *never, ever violate Rule 4*, as to do so may place a great burden not only on you, but on your loved ones (remember my Mexico story at the end of the last chapter).

Nutrition: Alternative or Supplement?

Let's start with wheat grass juice, shall we? Not too long ago, wheat grass juice was all the craze. In the gym, at the "natural juice" shop, on the grocery store "organic" shelf, wheat grass juice was everywhere. Some places would grow the little sprouts right there in front of you. You could watch them cut off a bunch of the bright green shoots, wash them, toss them into the blender, and voila, bright green wheat grass juice.

Now, I'm not saying that wheat grass juice doesn't contain some vitamins that might be good for you, cancer or not. Just that *on its own*, as a true alternative therapy (in violation of Rule 1), wheat grass juice has never cleared metastatic cancer cells out of a lymph node or put a single tumor into remission. Not everyone agrees with me (surprise!). One website enthusiastically exclaims, "If we look at oxygen as a bullet to kill cancer cells, then we should look at wheat grass as a shotgun blast at treating cancer. The number of ways it deals with cancer is incredible." Amazing. And to think that we still use chemotherapy, radiation, and surgery when all we need to do is recognize that grazing cows rarely die of cancer!

Listen, there are a lot of nutritional "supplements," "enzymes," "energizers," "antioxidants," and "supercharged therapies" being touted on the Internet as safe, side effect–free, alternative cures for cancer. So why am I picking on wheat grass juice? First of all, simply as an example to make my point about alternative therapies, and second, because of a personal experience with the wonder that is the wheat grass juice cancer cure.

I was practicing surgery in a large community hospital in San Diego when the call came from the Emergency Department. An airline traveler, soon after boarding a plane, had been asked by the flight attendants to disembark. Apparently the "acrid smell" arising from The Traveler had been so pungent that the passengers seated on either side (and even those in the rows in front and behind him) had complained within minutes of boarding.

Indeed, even before I opened the curtain surrounding his emergency room bed, I could clearly smell what those fellow passengers had smelled. Only unlike them, I knew what the smell was. It was the smell of decaying tissue, of a very large cancer long exposed to the air. The Traveler himself appeared in no distress, except for his obvious discomfort in sitting on the emergency room bed. He was an extremely thin gentleman (another giveaway that he harbored an advanced cancer) in his forties, well dressed, polite, and sad. He told me what had occurred only hours earlier on the airplane, and explained that the smell might have something to do with a small rectal cancer for which he had been receiving treatment.

On examination, The Traveler's "small rectal cancer" was an enormous tumor that protruded far out from his anus.

Enough of the unpleasant descriptives. Let's get back to wheat grass juice. The Traveler told me that he had first been diagnosed with the rectal cancer more than a year previously.

When told that the surgery recommended in an attempt to cure him would permanently leave him with a colostomy (wherein the end of the large intestine is brought through the abdominal wall and stool collects in a bag attached to the skin), he went searching for an alternative treatment option that still offered the true hope of cure without this drastic rerouting of his intestines. Early on in his search, he met the "nutritional doctor" who shared with The Traveler a history of successfully curing a variety of advanced tumors using—wait for it—wheat grass juice. This "doctor" shared numerous written testimonials from dozens and dozens of "incurable" cancer patients whose lives he had so safely and easily and comfortably saved, all without surgery, radiation, or chemo. So for the past year or so, The Traveler had paid thousands of dollars to the "nutritional doctor" in return for the curative "supercharged" wheat grass juice treatments. The Traveler, an otherwise rational man, had undergone an alteration in his mental evaluation processes, the very processes by which he had lived a successful professional and personal life, as a result of fear. The fear of his stool collecting in a colostomy bag attached to his skin under his shirt. He was unwilling to give up his shot at a cure, but the mental processes that had served him so well (and included a solid dose of skepticism) had been drastically altered by this fear.

And out of which third-world country did this wheat grass juice/snake oil salesman/nutritional doctor operate? What horrific, backward, unethical city produced such an evil charlatan? *Cleveland.*

The Traveler died under my palliative care less than a month later.

As I said, fear can be powerfully influential on all of us.

Wheat grass juice. "Nutritional doctor." "Supercharged therapies." "Enzymes" and "antioxidants" and "energetics." These and similar words and phrases should send up red flags and flashing red lights proclaiming, "CAUTION! LIKELY ALTERNATIVE THERAPY!"

So let's get to the facts. It is my informed opinion that nutritional supplements alone will not cure you or even slow the progression of your cancer. Nutritional supplements and the like should never serve as an alternative to the cancer treatments recommended to you by your cancer physicians.

However, nutrition does play a critical role in maximizing your potential to successfully battle your cancer and should be aggressively incorporated into your life *along with* your treatments, regardless of whether or not a cure is possible. Furthermore, nutritional challenges are common in those who harbor malignancies, as both the cancer itself and your treatments can alter your appetite and metabolism and sap you of your strength, stamina, and muscle mass. Every good cancer doctor and nurse and dietician knows this. And every good cancer doctor and nurse and dietician appreciates the importance that nutrition plays as a *supplemental* therapy in the treatment of cancer. So start by talking with your oncologist. If not offered, ask for (demand if necessary) to speak with a dietician, especially one who is interested in the important supplemental role nutrition plays for cancer patients. Ask questions, create lists, follow up with your dietician, and take charge, as your nutritional intake is one of the few critical treatments that *is* entirely under your control.

And as I've stated throughout this book, don't get your nutritional information off just any website that you happen to find, particularly those with claims that are too good to be true (they are). Rather, I encourage you to educate yourself about how to incorporate nutritional therapy into your own treatment regimen through such trustworthy websites as the American Cancer Society (Cancer.org), which has an excellent section on "Nutrition for People with Cancer," and the National Cancer Institute (Cancer.gov), which presents an "Overview of Nutrition in Cancer Care." Be smart and you'll find the guidance that will empower you to help yourself address your disease through the addition of nutritional therapy.

Your nutritional intake is one of the few critical treatments that is entirely under your control.

And remember, unlike all acceptable supplemental therapies, nutritional support stands alone in being critical in *every* cancer owner's fight against his or her malignancy.

And Acupuncture?

The American Cancer Society website (Cancer.org) best sums up the role that acupuncture, an ancient Chinese medical therapy wherein numerous thin needles are inserted through the skin to address disease and control symptoms, plays in the care of those suffering from cancer:

"Available scientific evidence does not support claims that acupuncture is an effective treatment for cancer. Still, it appears it may be useful as a complementary [supplementary] method for relieving some symptoms related to cancer and other conditions.

Acupuncture has been the subject of many clinical studies ... At this time, there is sound scientific support for acupuncture for 2 conditions: nausea/vomiting and headaches."

I've had patients who swear by acupuncture in reducing their nausea and vomiting, and others who felt that they gained nothing from the needles. The point to be made here is that if selected, acupuncture should be used *in addition* to your "Western" cancer treatments—that is, as a supplemental therapy. As such, remember that acupuncture is not a necessary treatment—it may or may not reduce or relieve symptoms—whereas nutritional supplemental therapy *is a must* in every cancer owner's treatment armamentarium.

Religiousness and Prayer

Not surprisingly, there is evidence that for many people receiving the diagnosis of cancer increases their "religiousness." If this is true for you (and/or a loved one), don't ever feel like a "fake" or "Johnny-come-lately." So many people in this world find God, religion, or spirituality for the first time when truly faced with a crisis. There is neither shame nor falseness in such an "awakening." Thus, if learning that you harbor a malignancy is what first brings you (or someone who loves you) religion, or if owning a cancer dramatically increases your spirituality, this is good. May it bring you comfort during this trying time in your life.

Prayer, in my experience, is unique among supplemental therapies. (Other than within a limited number of "extreme" religious groups, prayer is never offered or considered as an alternative therapy, a true replacement for standard medical treatment. The many, many proponents of prayer encourage its use in addition to accepted cancer therapies—that is, as a supplemental therapy.) Prayer may be rendered by the patient herself or himself or through "intercessory prayer" offered by loved ones and/or by others—even by total strangers.

Prayer offered by cancer owners themselves has yet to demonstrate objective clinical impact on their disease. Similarly, intercessory prayer, whether delivered by loved ones (a common event) or by people unknown or little known to the patient, while truly altruistic, has never clearly demonstrated an impact on clinical outcomes (such as survival). All that said, there is some evidence to suggest that intercessory prayer may make those for whom prayers are offered feel better "spiritually," which for some cancer patients may represent a significant benefit. And the mental, psychological, social, and spiritual benefits of prayers offered by loved ones and by cancer owners are hard to deny for any of us privileged to have shared in and/or witnessed the delivery of this deeply moving supplemental therapy. Many a time have I been humbled with an invitation from a patient or a spouse or a son or a daughter to bow my head as prayers are offered for the cancer owner. And the other times, truly solemn times, where I've stood back and witnessed the cancer-bearer alone, or the entire family, offering support and love through prayer just before I escorted the patient off to surgery. The effect on anyone observing, let alone participating in, such profound moments cannot help but to impart the acceptance that at the very least such efforts benefit the cancer patient and those who love him or her. So pray, if you are so inclined. Pray alone, pray with family, pray with friends. Agree and be thankful should others wish to pray for you, even if you are not a "praying person," as this demonstrates their love for you while simultaneously decreasing their feelings of impotence.

And feel free to pray for your physicians, nurses, and others with whom you have partnered in your cancer journey. Not infrequently have patients and family members asked for "my permission" in praying for me the day of or night before I take their loved one to the operating room. I am always awed by this and always thank them for doing so.

A Couple More Supplementals to Consider

We've already agreed to avoid all alternative therapies, as previously defined by the first three of the Four Rules, and to be cautious regarding supplemental therapies that drain your wallet (Rule 4). We have also discussed the vital role that supplemental nutritional therapy must play in every cancer owner's life, as well as the possible utility of acupuncture and the potential strength of prayer in supplementing your treatment. In addition to these reasonable supplemental treatments, we must add a few more:

Professional counseling (emphasis on *professional*) may be extremely beneficial to you and/or your family members. Remember, your loved ones are suffering as well. They're frightened too. Psychiatrists (who have the ability to prescribe antidepressants or other medications), psychologists, and others formally trained in the support of those facing health crises can be introduced to you and your family through your oncologist. Again, ask for this help

. . . there is no need for shame or embarrassment. And if you don't feel that you need such counseling for yourself, don't be critical or deter your wife or husband or daughter, son, or parent from reaching out for help. Encourage them. Again, they're struggling too.

Exercise is always a challenging supplemental therapy to discuss. Often more than the cancer itself, your treatments sap your energy and leave you exhausted. All you want to do is sleep (or, for many of you, throw up). What . . . not up for a game of tennis? A quick 5K? From your family and friends' perspective, seeing you like this is frightening. If only you would get up and take a walk down the street with them, *they'd* feel better (less frightened). Here's the truth. If you have the strength, then physical activity, even limited physical activity (like getting up and walking to the bathroom and then walking back to bed) is good for your body. It helps your heart. It helps your muscles. It helps your lungs. It helps your brain. You don't have to run a half marathon. Just do whatever you can. And *let your family and friends help you.* Let them support you by holding underneath your arm. Let them help guide you out of that chair. It will help you both. And ask your oncologist to introduce you to a physical therapist. These wonderful people can assess your situation and suggest and teach you and your family helpful exercises to perform at home.

Now It's Time to Wander Off the Reservation

"The Healing Touch" (touted by proponents as "a relaxing, nurturing energy therapy . . . [that] assists in balancing your physical, mental, emotional, and spiritual well-being . . . works with your energy field to support your natural ability to heal . . . and works in harmony with standard medical care"), "aura manipulation," astrology, and numerous other treatments are hawked all over the Internet (and on late-night cable) as supplemental therapies for a plethora of diseases, including cancer. I am not going to try to dissuade you from trying any of these, should they suit your fancy. And provided that they pass the Four Rules test.

Hell . . . who knows? Maybe a Sagittarius *doesn't* need chemo.

11

Talking About the Scary Stuff

You've invested time in reading this book and should now have a good grasp of what it means to claim ownership of and take the lead in decisions about your cancer. But I suspect it's not likely a question about cancer stages or various chemotherapy regimens that truly occupies your thoughts. So let's address the question: *What happens if my treatments fail?*

It's a fact. Cancer kills a lot of people every year. That said, a hell of a lot of people with cancer also survive every year, some who live with their cancer and others who have successfully defeated theirs. The two main factors that determine whether you are cured of your cancer, live for years with your cancer, or die from your cancer are your type of cancer and your stage at diagnosis. These two factors that ultimately control your destiny are almost all based on the luck of the draw rather than on any action or inaction on your part (aside from those of you who own a lung cancer after years of smoking, and I am not here to scold you but to help you, too). Now, many of you own cancer types and/or have earlier stage disease for which we have very successful treatments. Others of you have similarly curable cancer types, but your malignancies are already more advanced and have already spread, making your shot at cure far less certain. A handful of you reading this book pulled the shortest straw, owning a cancer and/or stage that we rarely succeed in curing. And on the other end of the spectrum, a small group of you have the "good" cancers, the ones that almost always present in an early stage and are almost always cured. But no matter which group you fall into, the truth is that *people with your type and stage of cancer have died as a result of their malignancies.*

Over the years, I've been privileged to hear and participate in discussions regarding death that have taken place between my patients and their families (and friends and clergy). And I've learned that our shared fear of death is based on an amazing variety of concerns. For example, many of my patients have been overwhelmed with fear and sorrow at the prospect of losing their life, of missing all of the joys that they regularly experienced and were planning to experience. Some of my deeply religious patients didn't actually fear "no longer being in this world," but they often feared that they were leaving their loved ones behind with financial constraints, or worried because they wouldn't be around to care for an aged parent. Fear of dying is both deeply personal and frequently composed of a number of different individual fears.

First of all, not admitting your fear benefits no one, and it worsens the stress both for you (although you may not believe it to be so) and certainly for those who love and care for you. Because you're not the only one who is scared that your cancer may kill you. And do you honestly think that they'll bring this up to you? I have repeatedly observed that sharing your fear of dying and allowing your loved ones to share their fear of your dying is a powerful and beneficial bonding experience, the importance and impact of which cannot be overstated. *Admitting your fear of dying from your cancer not only is not a weakness, it is a strength that will help you and your family and friends.* It is evidence of an honest and deep sense of self that opens the door for those who are suffering silently along with you because they love you. And don't just share your fear one time and then lock it away

Sharing your fear of dying and allowing your loved ones to share their fear of your dying is a powerful and beneficial bonding experience.

again inside your mental vault. Then again, don't go overboard and start every morning with, "What's for breakfast? Boy, am I famished! I sure am terrified that my prostate cancer is gonna kill me. French toast?"

Discuss your fear whenever it feels right to do so, and do your best to be open to hearing others tell you about their fear when it feels right for them. That said, it's both perfectly understandable and entirely reasonable to ask others to respect a "no cancer discussion" period of time, but do allow them to reopen the conversation later, preferably not much later; otherwise, they may never bring it up again, which is not what you want for those you love.

Once you're able to admit and share your fear of dying from your cancer, try to figure out the specific components that are driving that fear. There will be the obvious biggies, such as not being able to see your kids, hug your spouse, have a beer with your friends. But as an example, a common fear driver is worry that your death will mean that your spouse and family will face significant financial challenges and stress as they attempt to move on with their lives. Husbands or wives worry that should they die, their spouse may not have the money they need to pay the bills as they get older. Fathers or mothers worry that their absence and loss of income will significantly threaten their children's future, from keeping the house to paying for college, weddings, and so on. *The one action I have repeatedly witnessed that can dramatically reduce this financial fear is to discuss it with your spouse.* Share your money concerns with your wife or husband. Discuss your current finances, including together writing out and going over a list of all your savings, investments, debts, and other monetary situations. If complex, consider including a financial advisor in these discussions, first sharing your cancer diagnosis and then explaining that you are involving a professional because you want to best care for and protect your family in the event that your cancer is fatal. I have seen financial fears decrease greatly following these open, honest discussions. It's unlikely your spouse will initiate such a difficult talk, refusing to worry you with his or her financial stress when you are fighting for your very survival. So, cancer owner, *it falls to you to initiate such discussions.* And you will sleep so much better, as will your spouse, once you begin to face your financial fears through discussion, even if your talks don't produce solutions (although you'll be surprised how often you can craft solid action plans).

Also, speak with your spouse and work with your lawyer to update (or create) a will and other estate documents—find a recommended estate attorney if you don't yet have one. Putting these important processes and legal forms in place prior to your potential death allows you and your spouse to make certain that your affairs and inheritance are handled as you both wish. Don't leave this burden of estate planning to your spouse to deal with alone after your death. And when you do beat your cancer and survive, this important task will be done. Otherwise a sizable chunk of what you've earned will go to the US government—is that where you want your hard-earned money to go?

As with open discussions of your and your spouse's financial fears, you will find that speaking with your loved ones about other specific fears is of tremendous value. You (and they) may find that your fear decreases, that it occupies less of your mind's time, allowing you to enjoy more of your life. And again, these honest and emotional discussions, while draining, further strengthen the bonds you have with your friends and family regardless of whether any solutions are discovered. So talk about who will help your son learn to hit a curveball if you're not there. Figure out with your daughter who will help her choose her dress for her first prom if you can't. Try to listen and help your son when he talks about majoring in French literature. Assure your daughter that she will be a great scientist someday. Plan out who will move your mother into an assisted living facility when she can no longer live independently. Make sure your spouse knows that you believe in his or her ability to earn what's needed for the family if you are gone. Share with your loved ones whichever of these or similar fears are bouncing around in your head. Believe me, they have the same—and other—fears; they just don't want to "burden you" by bringing them up. So open the door for your closest loved ones to hear your fears and share theirs. Together, you'll find some solutions. And even when there are no solutions to be found, there is great strength for you all in the sharing.

All right, enough of sharing fears. Owning your cancer also means *sharing your pride, passion, joy, and love*. Every patient of mine who has openly and repeatedly told their loved ones of the things that make them proud, smile, and happy has clearly found that *sharing positives is the wonderful and unexpected silver lining to their dark cancer cloud*. We spoke of Sentinel Events very early on in this book. Recognizing within both positive Sentinel Events (marriages, births, graduations) and negative Sentinel Events (funerals, divorces, cancer) opportunities to tell those you love why and how much you care for them is a blessing. Everybody wins. I've seen fathers share their tremendous love for and pride in their now-adult children for the first time since those children were little kids . . . their sons and daughters hearing for the first time in decades their mom or dad's overpowering parental love for and pride in them. Tears flow, mouths smile, hugs ensue. Cancer, the malevolent driver of this process, is shoved to the background, making way for wonderful moments.

> *Sharing positives is the wonderful and unexpected silver lining to the dark cancer cloud.*

Lifesaving and Life-Sustaining Interventions: What's Right for You?

For those of you whose cancer type and/or stage already has significantly reduced your chance of ultimately surviving your disease, there is another group of common fears that you must own and share and discuss. First are the fears pertaining to physical suffering: your fear of pain, of difficulty breathing, and of other miserable afflictions at the hands of your disease. And in discussing these frightening things, you need to begin thinking about how you wish to approach the use of two related but slightly different interventions: life*saving* and life-*sustaining*. Again, these decisions are deeply personal and individual, so *never assume that even your spouse understands, let alone shares, your wishes for you.* Hell, many of us don't know ourselves what we would want when faced with such physical challenges until we are actually faced with them (and even then, our feelings may fluctuate). Talk with your spouse, your kids (if they're old enough), your friends, your spiritual advisor, whoever loves or cares for you and has an ear to listen to and a mouth to speak with you. And remember a couple of things. First of all, as long as you are awake and thinking clearly, *you can always change your mind about the role of medical intervention in your life.* For example, you may initially decide (with your family's input) that you don't wish to receive narcotics if you develop chronic pain, because you'll be damned if you're going to spend your final days and weeks with your family lost in a world of grogginess, sleep, and confusion. That's fine. Discuss your decision with your doctors and tell them that this is your wish and expectation. But should you develop debilitating pain that is not controlled with non-narcotic drugs, you absolutely can change your mind and ask for and receive narcotics. You're not under oath, here. And guess what? If you want, you can change your mind again and no longer use narcotics. It's your choice, and it's flexible. Just keep communicating your thoughts, fears, and decisions with your family and your physicians. And your physicians will support your decisions, even if they change regularly. Just keep them up-to-date.

What about interventions to keep you alive? As I alluded to, this complex area is often thought of as two related but differing processes: life*saving* and life-*sustaining* interventions. This seemingly subtle difference in terminology can be significant, and it is important that you understand the differences should you have cancer that ultimately leads to your death, or should you require such aggressive treatment to potentially cure you that the treatment itself may lead to life-threatening complications. A couple of examples may help to clarify the relative differences between lifesaving and life-sustaining treatments, allowing you to recognize that your wishes regarding each may also differ.

Let's say that during your chemo treatment, the potassium (an "electrolyte" salt) in your blood rises rapidly, as can happen when cancer cells die and rupture. If your potassium rapidly rises high enough, it can cause your heart to stop (cardiac arrest), which will kill you, cancer or no cancer. However, the medical intervention required to reverse your rising blood potassium and avert a cardiac death is safe, easy to administer, and works rapidly—you'll get intravenous fluid and a limited number of safe intravenous medications, and the threat will be negated within only a few hours as your blood potassium drops to normal levels. This is an example of a life*saving* intervention. It represents a short-term intervention that, if successful, saves your life and returns you to your immediate pre-emergency state. In this case, once your potassium is back to normal levels, you'll continue your chemo and, hopefully, move on toward a cure. The rise in potassium may never happen again, or it may occur with a future chemo treatment and again be rapidly, easily, and successfully addressed. *The intervention was performed to save your life and return you to your pre-emergency state.*

So it's a no-brainer to request that any and all life*saving* interventions are performed should you need one, right? Well, don't miss the key phrase hidden in my definition: *"return you to your pre-emergency state."* Hmmm . . . see where I'm going here? Even when the intervention is safe, simple, and rapid (as in this elevated blood potassium example), *it may not make sense to proceed with a lifesaving intervention based on your pre-emergency state.* I had a patient once, a wonderful woman in her seventies, who had widely metastatic malignant myeloma. She had been in and out of the hospital many times to treat the multiple, painful bone metastases that riddled her body. Always a joy to care for, she suffered greatly and complained rarely as we got to know each other over the months. During yet another hospitalization for pain control that was seemingly no different than any of the previous hospital admissions to treat her pain, my surgical team found her lying in her bed unconscious, unarousable, comatose. A rapid blood analysis revealed that she was suffering from extremely elevated blood calcium, the result of the widespread metastatic damage done to her bones. Treatment was simple, safe, and rapid (similar to the treatment of the high blood potassium we just discussed). *We didn't treat her*, even though saving her life would have been simple, safe, and taken only a few hours. Why not? She and I had discussed

209

on several occasions her wishes regarding lifesaving interventions, and "saving her life" simply to wake her up and "return her to her pre-emergency state" was not only something she had specifically made clear she did not want, it would have been a cruel action. Her pre-emergency state was one of chronic, severe, relentless pain requiring hospitalization after hospitalization, a painful quality of life that would only worsen until her inevitable death. So we left her alone to die painlessly in her sleep (which she did within a day), pain-free at last, and I was pleased that this was the final exit from our world for this wonderful woman.

So *determining whether you want to receive lifesaving intervention depends on your pre-emergency state*, including the likelihood that you are going to beat your cancer and an appreciation for what quality of life you are living and likely will be living in the near future with or without cancer.

That said, when asked by my patients, I routinely say that unless you are truly end-stage (in the final days or weeks of your life before your cancer wins) and/or unless you are in extreme misery (from pain, severe breathing difficulty, etc.) for which improvement (palliation) is unavailable, allowing for lifesaving intervention is a good idea. If it turns out it wasn't a good idea, once your life's been saved, tell 'em never to save you again.

Life-*sustaining* intervention is related, but different. By definition, life-sustaining intervention is intervention required for you to *continue living* (as opposed to being saved). Life-sustaining interventions are longer term than lifesaving interventions (some even permanently) and frequently carry their own associated risks once implemented. For most people, the simplest decision is to refuse life-sustaining actions that are *invasive*, will *dramatically reduce their quality of life*, and are *forever* (required for the remainder of their life). The classic example of such an often-refused life-sustaining intervention is placing a person permanently on a breathing machine ("ventilator dependence"). Now, the ventilator is one of the greatest medical inventions of the twentieth century. By placing people on ventilators for hours, days, weeks, or even months, these people can survive major surgical procedures that could not be successfully performed prior to the invention of breathing support systems (heart bypass surgery, lung surgery, liver transplant, many large cancer operations, and many, many more). People also no longer all die from pneumonia resulting in respiratory failure (the inability to breathe at a level required to live). Honestly, thank God for the ventilator. But these are all examples where the ventilator, while life-sustaining, is almost like an extended lifesaving intervention. Why? Because, again, the intervention is *not intended to be permanent* (or even long term) and *returns the heart-surgery or pneumonia patient to their very high-quality pre-emergency state*. Before his heart surgery, the ventilator-supported patient was a great father and a wonderful boss. Before her pneumonia, the ventilator-supported patient was a terrific elementary school teacher and friend. They had great lives and great futures, and the ventilator brings with it the expectation of a return to those great lives and great futures. But if you have terminal cancer, and your lung metastases have resulted in your inability to breathe in enough oxygen, and you're constantly gasping for breath and feeling like you're suffocating, placing you on a ventilator offers no promise of a return to a better life. In fact, you'll be on the ventilator until you die from your cancer—either you'll get pneumonia, which happens to very ill patients on ventilators, or your metastatic cancer will ultimately kill you. For many people, living their last days or weeks of life with a tube down their throat, requiring that they are heavily sedated so they don't gag, doesn't sound like the way to go.

But what if you're undergoing chemo and radiation treatment for your lung mets, and you and your doctors are very optimistic about how your treatment is going and expect that a reasonable quality and quantity of life still lie ahead of you, when in your weakened state you develop pneumonia? Don't you want to have your life sustained by a ventilator? In a couple of weeks, you'll hopefully be off the breathing machine and back to work attacking your cancer and enjoying your family. Thus each decision is unique, as each of your situations is different, and only you can incorporate all of the available current information and future quality- and quantity-of-life projections to determine what you want for you.

So *life-sustaining interventions can only promise a return to the life you had prior to the intervention*. Sound just like life*saving* interventions, don't they? Yes, they are similar. But again, the difference in my mind has always been that life-sustaining interventions are of longer or permanent duration and are frequently associated with potential complications themselves. The common theme here is fairly simple: If the lifesaving or life-sustaining intervention can return you to a life of a quality that to you is worth living, allow for this intervention. If, however, an intervention would return you to a quality of life that *to you* is no longer desirable (or even undesirable), tell your doctors that you don't want this intervention. Unfortunately, the decision is not always so clear-cut. The best approach is to discuss these things as fairly general topics with your loved ones and your physicians. Thus, my malignant myeloma patient didn't specifically refuse intervention to treat high blood calcium; she gave the broad directive not to take any action aimed at returning her to her current, painful state. For these discussions and decisions, you must depend heavily on your physicians' input, allowing them to explain what complications and emergencies are most likely to arise given your specific cancer situation and the potential duration and risks associated with those most likely interventions. Such discussions shared ahead of any emergency event allow you, your family, and your doctors to take emergency lifesaving or life-sustaining actions, should they be indicated, or to *not* take emergency actions, based on an appreciation for *what you want*. And one discussion just won't cut it. You should revisit your thoughts and decisions as your treatment progresses (with favorable or unfavorable progress) and as your cancer status changes (for better or worse) and as your current and future anticipated quality of life changes (improves or diminishes). I know these are scary topics to consider and talk about, but owning them is part of owning your cancer and, as a result, owning the remainder of your life.

One more thing. Regardless of cancer type and stage, all of you should make certain that you have an up-to-date **advance directive.** An advance directive, often called a "living will," is a legal form that is simple to create and explains your wishes regarding what actions should be taken to care for you should you no longer be capable of making decisions regarding your health care. An advance directive can also empower another specific individual to make all decisions regarding your health care should you be unable to make decisions for yourself. The forms may differ from state to state and the language updated periodically, so be sure to ask your doctor for help in obtaining the right one for you. Just as important, make sure that the hospital has a copy of your most recent advance directive in the front of your hospital chart. And make sure that the doctors and nurses who care for you during any and every planned and/or emergency hospital admission know that you have an advance directive in your chart. Tell your family, too, in case they need to convey this information for you. The number of patients who do not have an advance directive is ridiculously high. Worse yet, many who do have advance directives fail to provide a copy to the hospital when they are admitted. More unbelievable is how often I have met patients who both had an advance directive and had provided a copy to the hospital upon admission, but the advanced directive was nowhere to be found in their chart. Finally, there are the patients who have an advance directive and have provided a copy to the hospital upon admission and who have a copy in the front of the chart, but whose doctors and nurses have no idea whether their patient has an advance directive when the question first arises during an emergency . . . Sorry. *It's still all on you*, cancer owner.

Now don't get me wrong. Having an advance directive does not replace sharing your health care wishes with your loved ones, particularly your spouse. The more your husband or wife truly appreciates *your wishes* (which may be very different from *their wishes for you*), the better for you should you become incapable of making decisions regarding your own care, and the better for them (as you have dramatically lessened their burden of guessing what you would want). Advance directive. Open discussions with your spouse and doctors ahead of time. Do it. Own it.

How Does Cancer Kill You?

Now that you have a basic yet meaningful understanding of tumor growth and spread, and a foundational appreciation of the various treatments that you may be offered, and you are clear on the meaning of "cure" and "survival" and "recurrence," let's discuss a difficult topic: If you lose your battle with your cancer, how does your cancer kill you? First, remember that many cancer patients are cured of their disease, living long, productive lives after completing their treatment. This is important to say, as many of you reading this book will (thankfully) beat your cancer; it's just that you might not know at this time if you're one of those cancer survivors. And some of you may already know or strongly believe that you are not.

Death from cancer most commonly results from metastatic disease, either present at the time of your initial diagnosis or, more frequently, recognized later as recurrent disease following treatment that was aimed at curing you. Persistent local disease or recurrent local cancer (both occurring at the primary tumor site) can also eventually kill you, although this is a less common scenario than death due to metastatic malignancy.

Whether metastatic, local, persistent, or recurrent, cancer most commonly leads to death through one of two pathways. Metastatic disease commonly overwhelms the organ in which it is growing, leading to failure of the organ—meaning that the invaded organ is unable to adequately continue the critical life-sustaining functions it has performed your entire life. For example, dozens of cancer mets within a person's lungs can limit the lungs' ability to bring in fresh oxygen and release carbon dioxide, often the result of a massive buildup of fluid around the lungs in response to the cancer mets themselves or the result of collapse of lung tissue distant to breathing tubes blocked by malignant growths. A heavy "cancer burden" in the liver (that is, numerous and/or large cancer mets) can result in the failure of the liver to perform one or more of its crucial functions, also leading to death. These two examples are typical scenarios by which cancer patients die as a result of their metastatic disease impeding critical life functions.

While less common a cause of death, critical organ failure can also result from primary site malignancy (persistent local disease or recurrent cancer). A primary lung tumor can damage the lung, leading to infections and obstructed breathing. A large colon cancer can suddenly perforate (create a hole in the large bowel), potentially leading to a rapid death. Such primary site-induced organ compromise is more likely palliated or prevented with a procedure or surgery than is organ failure due to widely metastatic disease. Thus, the failure of normal bodily functions as a result of cancer (usually metastatic, but occasionally primary) is one of the common ways in which cancer leads to the death of its owner. Whether such a death is "comfortable" or not depends in large part on the organ system that is failing as a result of the malignant disease. Many would find dying from kidney or liver failure vastly preferable (more comfortable) than dying from respiratory (lung) failure or intestinal perforation. As discussed previously, these are important differences to consider when thinking about lifesaving and life-sustaining interventions, should your cancer be incurable.

The other common manner in which cancers kill their owners is by "stealing their strength." Whether persistent or recurrent, advanced cancer (most often widely metastatic disease but occasionally the result of a very large primary tumor) changes the patient's body into one that mimics that of a prisoner of war. The person rapidly loses weight, their muscles and fat disappearing over weeks and months, their eyes "sinking in." The process producing this deterioration in "body habitus" is called **cancer cachexia.** Cachectic patients are weak, easily fatigued, and sleep much or most of the day and night. While this is difficult for a loved one to view, fortunately, many of these folks are relatively pain-free. They're just totally exhausted, severely nutritionally depleted, and fading fast, all the result of yet another horrific cancer characteristic: Cancer cells secrete proteins that trigger the breakdown of the patient's normal skeletal muscles and fat deposits. Thus while small overall in comparison to the remainder of the body, the tumor or tumors can trigger the loss of as much as 80 percent of a patient's skeletal muscle and fat. In addition, cancer cachexia often produces anorexia, and this significant loss of appetite only compounds the tremendous loss of muscle and fat, leading to "wasting" that seems to occur right before the very eyes of the patient's loved ones. It is reasonably argued that cancer cachexia (which some think of as "total body failure") is a preferable way to die, as many patients are simply asleep for most of their final days, often without any pain or significant breathing difficulty. Many simply pass away due to cardiovascular (heart) failure. Having shared in this part of the journey several times, I agree with this perspective: Most of my cancer cachexia patients were relatively or completely pain-free, were not struggling to breathe, and were just "tired out." They simply wished to go to sleep, which ultimately they did, forever.

These two journeys to death, organ failure and cancer cachexia, are not mutually exclusive. Many patients become cachectic because their organs are harboring dozens of growing cancer metastases that, in addition to secreting the cachexia proteins, are impeding critical bodily functions. Thus, for many cancer patients, the actual cause of death is the combination of rapid body mass loss compounding and compounded by increasing organ failure. Ultimately, the exact cause of death doesn't really matter. What does matter is doing everything possible to make their passing as pain-free and free of respiratory struggles as possible, even if the provision of drugs necessary to do so keeps these individuals asleep for most of their remaining time. Keeping terminal patients as comfortable as possible is the goal of hospice and palliative care, and seeking such professional assistance is often the best approach for patients and loved ones.

Again, remember: *Many if not most of you reading this book will not die of your cancer*. Sadly, however, some of you will, and a few of you no doubt know right now, from speaking with your doctors, that cure is a long shot, or perhaps not even possible. For all of you, regardless of which group you ultimately fall into, it is important to address how cancer death occurs, because it's been on your mind (and on the minds of those who love you). You've thought about it (even by trying *not* to think about it). And in order to own your cancer, you must ask the tough questions and hear the hard answers, allowing you to better understand and guide yourself down your ultimate pathway.

12

You May Not Like Your Relatives, But You Should Help Them

A very short chapter on yet another action that you as a cancer owner must initiate to help other people. (Who knew that being diagnosed with cancer would mean you would have to become even more responsible for helping other people?) We have learned a great deal about how and why several of the more common cancers develop. Some arise through spontaneous carcinogenesis, meaning that as of today, we have not identified any environmental factors (that is, anything that you did) or genetic factors (that is, anything that Mom or Dad passed on to you) that played a direct role in the development of that specific type of cancer. We know of a handful of non-spontaneous cancers that arise *in association with environmental factors*. Lung cancer is far and away the most environmentally associated common cancer, developing in the overwhelming majority of patients as a direct result of their smoking. And more recently we have begun identifying more and more *genetic links* to different cancers.

Understanding any relationships between our individual genetic profiles and the risk of cancer development is a challenging and exciting new field that truly will lead to "personalized medicine." Each and every cell in our body contains DNA, the instruction manual for our development from conception to death. Our DNA instruction manual is written in segments called genes. Together, our approximately 25,000 genes serve to determine our hair color, our height, our myriad liver functions, our intelligence, our heart rate, our kidney function, and everything else that contributes to making each one of us who we are as individuals. Our genes also control the functions of every cell in our body (including cell growth and programmed cell death). When certain genes or combinations of genes no longer work correctly, the tasks governed by those genes may no longer work correctly. Errors in how genes instruct the cells of our body to function are called **mutations.** Mutations can be inherited from one or both parents or can occur when our normal cells are replicating (copying themselves and then dividing into two cells). We are finding ever more gene profiles (the presence or absence of activity in individual genes or combinations of genes) that are associated with measurable increases in the risk of cancer development. Two genes, BRCA1 and BRCA2, are linked to breast cancer in both women and men and to ovarian cancer in women. The normally functioning BRCA1 and BRCA2 genes are not associated with increased cancer risk and, in fact, are important in regulating normal cell growth. However, errors in correctly copying normal DNA can occur as cells are replicating and dividing, resulting in BRCA1 and/or BRCA2 gene mutations. Such a genetic mutation can be passed on to offspring, and inheriting a mutated BRCA1 or BRCA2 gene results in an elevated risk of breast and ovarian cancer once the child becomes an adult. In the general population of women who have inherited normal BRCA1 and BRCA2 genes, the risk of developing breast cancer is about 12 percent. Inherit a BRCA1 or BRCA2 mutation, however, and your risk of breast cancer rises to a whopping 60 percent. That's **genetic susceptibility** to breast cancer. At least 5 percent of all colon and rectal cancers are a result of hereditary nonpolyposis colorectal cancer (HNPCC), an inherited syndrome that predisposes you not only to colon and rectal cancers, but also cancers of the uterus, ovary, intestines, and urinary tract. In HNPCC, genetic mutations are inherited and are present in every cell of a person's body. The normal (non-mutated) genes play an important role in repairing DNA when errors occur during copying (cell replication); that is, the normal genes allow cells to create the proteins necessary to repair critical DNA copying errors, protecting us from the dangers of mutations. When the mutation-repairing genes themselves are mutated, they no longer function, making it much more likely that DNA replication errors will persist within cells, resulting in a much greater potential for cancer development.

We have identified the genes responsible for the HNPCC syndrome. Like the BRCA1 and BRCA2 gene mutations, many HNPCC gene mutations can frequently be identified through simple blood tests. These are but two examples of the numerous already identified genetic abnormalities that are associated with the development of different cancers. And the list keeps growing as we learn more and more about our **genome** (the collection of all of our 25,000 or so genes). Even in the absence of specific genetic understanding, we know of many cancers that have a hereditary element; that is, your likelihood of developing the cancer is increased if your mother, father, and/or sibling had the same (or sometimes a different) type of cancer.

Your oncologist can tell you whether your cancer history, your family's cancer history, and especially your type of cancer may mean that your first-degree relatives (your biological mother, biological father, biological children, and biological siblings) are also at a higher risk of developing the same or a different cancer. If your cancer has or may have developed as a result of such a known inherited risk, then *you can literally save the life of your child, brother, sister, and/or parent* by making them aware of their risk and thus potentially preventing cancer development or catching a cancer at a treatable stage.

I will never forget one wonderful patient. He was a compassionate man, loving husband, and successful author. Because he was only in his forties when first referred to me with a newly diagnosed colon cancer, I was immediately suspicious that his malignancy was a result of the inherited genetic syndrome we discussed, HNPCC. He had many of the hallmarks of the syndrome, including his young age, cancer location, and family history of certain cancers in young relatives. His parents had both passed away, but he and his equally wonderful and impressive wife had one son who was in his early twenties. Their son was, understandably, struggling greatly with the situation (his father, my patient, had advanced cancer when we first met), and their time together was often spent in uncomfortable silence or jagged small talk. I spoke with my patient about "owning his cancer," and soon he was initiating conversations, telling his son how proud he was of the man he had become and how much he loved the boy. It took a little while, but things certainly did change. The two of them began regularly talking honestly and comfortably, even about uncomfortable topics. And finally, the most uncomfortable topic came up. As relayed to me by my very happy patient only weeks before he died, his son began crying, telling his dad that he couldn't handle his impending death. The father smiled warmly, tears flowing down his cheeks, and told his son, "At least through my death, I might save you." He had convinced his son to undergo the genetic testing that could identify the presence of the genetic mutations associated with HNPCC, genes indicating an elevated risk that his son would also develop potentially fatal colon cancer at a young age. His son was positive for the mutated genes; he did indeed carry the risk. And just before my patient died, he expressed overwhelming joy when his son told him that during a screening colonoscopy (when I used a scope to look into the son's large intestine) I had removed a benign growth that likely would have become a cancer within less than a decade. His son assured his dying father that he would undergo these simple colonoscopy procedures every five years for the rest of his life. Having any pre-cancerous growths removed meant his son would never get (let alone die from) colon cancer. Truth be told, all three of us were crying as we stood in that hospital room, all of us realizing that the older-yet-still-so-young father had truly likely protected his son from a similar early fate and, in fact, had further helped protect his yet unborn grandchildren. What a gift my friend gave his boy just before leaving us.

But *I* could not have convinced my patient's son to get the genetic testing, let alone undergo a colonoscopy. It is *you* who have the greatest influence on your relatives. You who will be the most successful in convincing them to have simple genetic screening tests. Tell them about how your cancer can be inherited and thus how your having cancer suggests that they, too, might carry the inherited risk of malignancy. Have your doctor help you in discussing this and in explaining how and what genetic screening tests are available and what the potential outcomes suggest. Tell them you love them and are asking that they learn from your situation and that they protect themselves from having to go through what you're going through.

You'll be surprised by how many of your relatives will push back or clearly deny or ignore what you're saying. Because *they'll be scared*. So be compassionate (again, you, the cancer owner, have to be the compassionate one). Don't expect a "Yes, right away!" answer. After all, just minutes before, it was *your* cancer. Now you and a guy in a white coat are telling them it may also be *their* cancer risk. The fact that you're only telling them of the *possibility* that they may potentially also share genetic mutations associated with a higher risk of cancer development *some day* is irrelevant . . . you're scaring the living crap out of them! Give them time to absorb it all. Stop the discussion when they clearly need a break. But don't let the topic drop off the radar. Follow up. Ask on a subsequent visit if they have scheduled an appointment with a doctor to move forward with their genetic screening. If they haven't, be patient. Ask again in a couple of days (if they don't visit or call you, *you* visit or call them). If they are still hedging or outright refusing (denial mixed with fear is a powerful driver of illogical inaction), change it from your recommendation to *your expectation*. Hell, even demand it. Here's your chance to play the "cancer card," to use guilt as someone "suffering from cancer" to press a relative into granting you one simple request, to do you this one simple favor that will make you happy (and, by the way, which may save their friggin' life). Recruit their spouse or other relatives and friends, if necessary. *Just make it happen.*

Now, if your doctor suggests that you do likely have an inherited (genetic-based) cancer, you likely don't need to press all of your relatives to be screened, just your first-degree relatives. These include your biological children, biological siblings, and biological parents. I have noticed that getting your children to be screened to prevent their developing your cancer tends to be the least challenging, as they seem to be acutely impacted by what's happening to their once seemingly invincible mom or dad and are often in the midst of preparing for the joys of their own long lives. Siblings can be a pain to convince, as there always seems to be at least one brother or sister who chronically denies and provides excuses. Stay on 'em. Parents are often the most difficult, at least at first. If your cure is unlikely or impossible, your parents will likely struggle as they believe that they should die before you, their child, dies. Or they feel overwhelming guilt for having cursed you with a cancer that arose from mutations inherited from them (genetically speaking, they're right, but transforming such an inheritance into a preventable, malicious act is nonsensical, as no genetic testing was available for them). Thus, parents often shrug off the request to undergo screening to protect them from your cancer or cancer syndrome. However, with parents you have leverage that simply does not exist when pressing your siblings or children: guilt. Use it as necessary, even liberally, if that's what it takes to get your sixty-eight-year-old mother to be evaluated. "What? *You don't want to go to your granddaughter's wedding* some day? *You're willing to die from a preventable cancer just because I have cancer?*" You'll win. And why the hell shouldn't your mother live another ten years?

13

What About Sex? Living with Cancer

It's an odd, even surreal thing, really. I mean, think about it (I'm sure you have). You were living your life, year after year, month after month, week after week, day after day. You were going to work or watching the grandkids. You were paying your electric bill and shopping for groceries. You were still putting off taking the car in even though the "Check Engine" light had been on for a month. You were out of underwear but hadn't done the laundry. You were reheating the extra Kraft Mac & Cheese. And when you had that rare moment alone with your beloved, and you weren't actually too damn tired, you made love with your wife or husband. Month after month, week after week, day after day. You were a person living your life.

That was only yesterday (or just last week or last month). In a flash, you were no longer a "person." No, you suddenly and completely were a "patient." A "cancer patient." One minute you were a person sitting in the exam room, waiting for the doctor to come in (perhaps anxiously, perhaps not). Literally the next minute, it all changed. "It's cancer." "You've got cancer." Whatever the words, it didn't matter—when you've been hit by a truck, it doesn't matter how many wheels the truck has.

That's the weird thing about cancer. When you think back on all the Sentinel Events in your life (as we discussed way back at the beginning of this book), you realize that cancer is fairly unique in its suddenness. I mean, you have an inkling that you're going to marry your longtime girlfriend or boyfriend. And for God's sake, you have nine months to stress over the joys of parenthood. Even divorce rarely comes as a sudden surprise. But cancer . . . well, you may have been feeling a bit out-of-sorts for a few weeks, and you may even have worried, at least just a little, with the "C word" slipping in and out of your thoughts. But you didn't really believe it was true. And many of you either felt minimally ill (as you have dozens of times during your life) or felt totally fine and were simply undergoing your annual physical exam and blood tests. So for many of you, hearing "you have cancer" was sudden, hitting you and your loved ones like the proverbial ton of bricks.

In fact, the only other Sentinel Event that on occasion similarly strikes us down out of the blue is . . . death. The ringing phone in the early morning hours. The sudden, overwhelming shock. Again, surreal.

So like the unexpected or relatively rapid death of a loved one or friend, one minute you're a person living your life, and the next minute you're a cancer patient, living your cancer patient life. . . .

The choice is yours. I have seen many a person "throw in the towel," accept their new cancer patient identity, and passively move through their surgery and radiation and chemotherapy and CAT scans and blood tests as if already dead. And some of these people turn out in the end of it all to survive their cancer. Again, no blame here . . . understanding and sympathy all around for those who have accepted this passive role. But *don't you do it*.

Own it, damn it. Own your damn cancer. Own it. Don't allow all of your life's experiences, all of your relationships, all of your joys and challenges, all of your skills and knowledge, don't allow all of this priceless information to get filed away in the "no longer of use" cabinet by accepting the label of "cancer patient." *Screw that*. Unless you are unable, take out the garbage on garbage night (and if you are unable, asking your son or daughter to take out the garbage still allows you to participate in your and their lives, as you have your entire adult life). Pick up some Chinese food for the family. Maybe you don't eat it if you're still nauseated from your chemo, but pick it up and sit with your loved ones while the mushrooms slip out of their chopsticks. Go to a movie if you can, and if you can't, sit on the couch with your friend and watch one on cable (no big deal if you doze off, tired from your radiation). And for God's sake, make love to your partner. You've got cancer, but you're not made of fine crystal. You're not going to break, and you sure as hell can't give your spouse your disease. Lost some of your hair? I think he'll still sleep with you (you were having sex with him long after he got that larger belly).

"Cancer patients" are owned by their cancers. "People with cancer" own their cancers and continue to live their lives.

Too exhausted to make love? Then fondle and kiss and cuddle. Still too much only one day after radiation? Then just look him or her in the eye and say, "I sure as hell love you" (and feel free to add, "Once I've licked this thing, you better run . . . fast!").

"Cancer patients" are owned by their cancers. "People with cancer" own their cancers and continue to live their lives, as different as those lives need to be. The reality is, other than the short-term limitations on certain physical activities in the weeks immediately following your surgery, there is truly nothing significant that you are medically prohibited from doing simply because you happen to have cancer or are undergoing treatment for cancer. *You are just a person continuing to live your life and, at this time, your life includes your owning a cancer.* And still owning and caring for your dog. And still grilling (and burning) burgers. And dealing with your cranky neighbor. And your lovely daughter. And your beater car.

So that's it. That's all I got. It's your time to once again step up and take control, as you have so many times throughout your life. Learn whatever you need to learn, ask whatever you need to ask (again and again, if necessary). Keep living your life despite the frightening thoughts and anxious moments that will frequently barge in, pulling you away from your friends and family, seeking to take you down dark mental pathways for long periods of time. Just come back to your loved ones as soon as you can and return to your life, in all its glory. After all, pipes break in houses and car engines fail, but we move on, because we love our homes and our cars. That's what "ownership" means.

14

So Now You Know . . .

No one doctor can possibly know all there is to know about cancer. Hell, no one doctor can know all there is to know about *thyroid* cancer, let alone all cancers. Or everything there is to know about radiation treatments. Or all of the side effects of all the chemotherapy agents.

Nor can any one person with cancer.

But as a person with cancer, or as a loved one of a person with cancer, you don't even need to know a fraction of all that your doctors actually do know. You do, however, need to know two things.

First, you must possess a basic understanding of the medical concepts and processes and the personal challenges that are critical to addressing your cancer. These are the varied topics that we've discussed in this book (which you have successfully completed, and I'm proud of you). With this knowledge, you will maximize your involvement in decisions that directly impact your future, and you will minimize your exclusion from your life as you deal with your malignancy, whether you are ultimately successful or whether you ultimately die from your cancer.

The second and final thing you need to know is something that is known only to you. That is, what do you want out of the rest of your life? "The rest of your life" includes this current, horrific period that is focused on your disease. Yet whether or not your cancer ultimately kills you, *you must not allow "the rest of your life" to be completely or permanently defined by your malignancy.* If you have the strength and commitment, take everything that you know to be true about yourself and are willing to honestly share with yourself and combine it with the knowledge that you've garnered from this book. If you can do this, you will possess a foundation of insight and understanding that will truly empower you now and for "the rest of your life," regardless of how long that is. And that, my friend, will mean that you are in the purest and most universal sense *the owner of your cancer.*

I wish you a wonderful life.

— Dr. E

Appendix

Finding the Right Cancer Physician Partners

If you truly own your cancer, you must search for and find cancer physicians who are the right "fit" for you. Not only should your physician partners be experienced and knowledgeable, they must also complement your personality and demonstrate an interest in developing a relationship with you and your loved ones. Following are some basic questions to help you find the right cancer surgeon, radiation oncologist, and medical oncologist partners. It is important that you not only listen to the *substance* of what they tell you, but also to the *tone* and *style* of their answers. Is the physician confident? Arrogant? Too serious? Not serious enough? Does the physician make certain that you and your loved ones clearly understand what he/she is saying? Does the physician sound interested? Distracted? Intelligent? Are you encouraged to ask questions? Is the physician patient? Too young? Too old? Pay attention and trust your instincts—you know yourself, and this will help you successfully identify doctors whose tone, style, and personality match your needs. If they are also experienced and knowledgeable, you've found your cancer physician partners. I appreciate that what insurance you have, where you live, and other real-world factors impact what doctors are available to care for you. That said, if you have any physician options, these questions will help you find the better "fit" doctors for you. And if after pushing hard to have a choice you still have no physician options, these questions will empower you to understand your doctors and their approach to your care.

Questions you should ask when trying to determine if a SURGEON is the right "fit" for you:

1. **What to Ask:** "How much training did you receive in treating patients with my type and stage of cancer?"
    Why It Matters: General surgical training often provides adequate experience in the treatment of common types and stages of cancer. For less common types and more advanced or complex malignancies, you should seek out a *fellowship-trained surgeon*. Following general surgical training, fellowship training often provides additional experience in treating less common and more advanced cancers. (If you are fortunate and have a fellowship-trained surgeon near you, meet that surgeon even if your cancer is one of the more common types.)

2. **What to Ask:** "How frequently in your current practice do you treat people with my type and stage of cancer?"
    Why It Matters: In surgical cancer care, experience counts, and you will depend heavily on your surgeon's knowledge and professional experience. You want to partner with a surgeon who regularly cares for cancer owners like you (both in type and stage).

3. **What to Ask:** "What will you remove during surgery in addition to my tumor?"

Why It Matters: It is important to understand what normal body tissues the surgeon would remove along with your tumor and what impact this loss will have on your body's function in both the short and long term. Also, you must understand the surgeon's plan regarding removal of lymph nodes, a critical part of virtually all cancer operations. Look for a surgeon who demonstrates experience, confidence, patience, and the ability to clearly explain things.

4. **What to Ask:** "Are there treatments other than the one you are recommending?"

   Why It Matters: For some types and stages of cancer, there are different approaches to treatments which include surgery (for example, radiation may be used before, during, or after surgery). You want a surgeon who is knowledgeable in all methods used to treat your type and stage of cancer. You also want a surgeon with the experience and confidence to recommend a specific treatment approach.

5. **What to Ask:** "Who will assist you during my operation?"

   Why It Matters: In most operations, the surgeon is assisted by at least one other surgeon or certified assistant. In teaching hospitals, surgeons are routinely assisted by surgical interns and residents (medical doctors training to be surgeons) and/or by medical students. Knowing who will assist the surgeon and their roles in the operation and in your post-operative care may influence your decision (favorably or unfavorably) regarding that surgeon.

Questions you should ask when trying to determine if a RADI-ATION ONCOLOGIST is the right "fit" for you:

1. **What to Ask:** "How frequently in your current practice do you treat people with my type and stage of cancer?"
   Why It Matters: Experience counts in the complex delivery of radiation therapy. Partnering with a radiation oncologist who routinely treats your cancer type and stage will likely increase the benefits and reduce the risks associated with your radiation treatment.

2. **What to Ask:** "Will I always be cared for by you, or will other radiation oncologists in your group see me?"
   Why It Matters: You may receive radiation before, during, and/or following surgical treatment. Thus, your radiation oncologist is truly your partner for months. Radiation is also used to help lessen pain and other symptoms associated with recurrent and incurable tumors (such as metastatic bone pain). For both curative and palliative care, working with a single radiation oncologist who knows you and your cancer history greatly helps in gauging and adjusting your treatment to fit your shared goals.

3. **What to Ask:** "Is there more than one way to deliver radiation to treat my type and stage of cancer?"
   Why It Matters: There are many types of expensive and complex equipment and methods to deliver radiation to tumors. Each delivery method has its own potential benefits (more

radiation hitting the tumor) and risks (damage to healthy tissues surrounding the cancer). A radiation oncologist whose treatment recommendation is based solely on what equipment and delivery system is available in his or her office is not the right partner for you. It is critical to find a radiation oncologist who is knowledgeable about treatment options and is recommending a radiation delivery plan that seeks to maximize the benefits and minimize the risks specific to treating *you*.

4. **What to Ask:** "What will be the short- and long-term effects of this radiation treatment on my body?"
   Why It Matters: Radiation therapy routinely injures the normal, healthy tissues surrounding the targeted tumor. It is not uncommon for the injured tissues to bleed, cause pain, or produce other symptoms. Depending on what part of your body was radiated and how the radiation was delivered, some of these problems last only weeks or months while others may affect you for the rest of your life. An experienced, honest, and communicative radiation oncologist will clearly explain these risks so that you can understand the potential problems you may face.

5. **What to Ask:** "How often and for how long will I receive radiation treatment?"
   Why It Matters: Radiation therapy is often the most logistically challenging part of your cancer treatment. It is routinely delivered in a sequence of brief daily sessions for several days, followed by a couple of days off, with this cycle repeating for

several weeks. Thus radiation therapy can be a real transportation challenge for you and your loved ones (the vast majority of radiation patients need others to drive them). Understanding up front the treatment time commitment allows you and your support network to adequately plan for all the back-and-forth driving.

Questions you should ask when trying to determine if a MEDICAL ONCOLOGIST is the right "fit" for you:

1. **What to Ask:** "How frequently in your current practice do you treat people with my type and stage of cancer?"
   Why It Matters: There are thousands of types and stages of cancer, chemotherapy drugs, and combinations of chemo drugs. As a result, medical oncologists routinely treat a wide variety of malignancies but most truly focus on a limited number of cancers. Given that this will likely be the physician with whom you partner the longest, it is essential that you find an oncologist who is experienced, passionate, and focused on the treatment of your specific type of cancer.

2. **What to Ask:** "How many chemotherapy regimens (drug combinations) can be used to treat my type and stage of cancer?"
   Why It Matters: There may be more than one chemo regimen (combination of chemo drugs) that can be used to treat your cancer type and stage because sometimes there is no

one clearly superior regimen. Each regimen offers unique benefits and risks. You should partner with an oncologist who possesses both significant knowledge of all chemotherapy options for you and the experience to support a specific recommendation.

3. **What to Ask:** "If this chemotherapy regimen is not working, will we switch to another?"

   Why It Matters: The success of a chemo regimen varies even in people with similar cancers. Experienced oncologists have milestones to determine the effectiveness of chemo treatment. Ask the oncologist how the effectiveness of the chemo regimen is determined, how often the regimen fails for your type and stage of cancer, and what the oncologist does (changes doses, changes drugs) when the chemotherapy is not working.

4. **What to Ask:** "What are the most common and the most dangerous side effects of the chemo treatment you are recommending?"

   Why It Matters: Chemo commonly causes side effects that range from mild to miserable. However, the most common side effects often are not the most dangerous ones. Knowing what you are likely to experience prepares you and your loved ones, and understanding the most dangerous possibilities tells you what to look for so that you can immediately seek help should symptoms develop.

5. **What to Ask:** "Are there any clinical trials for people with my cancer type and stage?"

   Why It Matters: The majority of clinical trials test new chemotherapy drugs on patients whose cancer cannot frequently be cured using standard treatments. However, some clinical trials enroll people with more curable cancers, offering new chemo drugs in addition to (not instead of) standard chemo treatment. It never hurts to ask if you qualify to enroll in a clinical trial and if you do, to investigate further.

Resources

The list below includes resources mentioned in this book. I've also included three patient support organizations and a comprehensive cancer center for children suffering from cancer (identified by ♦ bullets) that I did not mention in the book. *This is not an exhaustive list* of great and credible institutions and foundations; that is, there are many others that you can rely on in addition to those offered here.

American Cancer Society (while a national organization, the American Cancer Society also has many regional and local chapters): cancer.org

City of Hope Cancer Center (Duarte, California): cityofhope .org

Cleveland Clinic (Cleveland, Ohio): my.clevelandclinic.org

Clinical Trials Registry & Results Database (a service of the US National Institutes of Health): ClinicalTrial.gov

Dana-Farber Cancer Institute (Boston, Massachusetts): dana-farber.org

Duke Cancer Institute (Durham, North Carolina): DukeCancer Institute.org

Johns Hopkins (Sidney Kimmel Comprehensive Cancer Center, Baltimore, Maryland): hopkinsmedicine.org

♦LIVESTRONG Foundation (founded by cancer survivor Lance Armstrong, this group provides support to patients, raises funds for research, and serves as a forum and voice for cancer patients): livestrong.org

Massachusetts General Hospital Cancer Center (Boston, Massachusetts): massgeneral.org

Mayo Clinic Cancer Center (the main Mayo Clinic is in Rochester, Minnesota, but Mayo Clinics are also in Phoenix and Scottsdale, Arizona, and in Jacksonville, Florida): MayoClinic.org

MD Anderson Cancer Center (Houston, Texas): mdanderson .org

Memorial Sloan-Kettering Cancer Center (New York City): mskcc.org

Moffitt Cancer Center (Tampa, Florida): moffitt.org

National Cancer Institute: cancer.gov

♦St. Jude Children's Research Hospital (the first and only National Cancer Institute–designated Comprehensive Cancer Center that is devoted solely to children. Memphis, Tennessee): stjude.org

♦Stand Up 2 Cancer (a terrific national organization that provides support to patients, raises funds for research, and serves as a forum and voice for cancer patients): standup2cancer.org

Stanford Cancer Institute (Palo Alto, California): cancer.stanford.edu

♦Stupid Cancer ("The Voice of Young Adults Affected by Cancer" is a nonprofit organization that provides innovative and award-winning programs and services for this unique subset of adult cancer patients): StupidCancer.org

Index

About the Author

Dr. Peter Edelstein, MD, FACS, FASCRS, is a double–board certified physician with years of experience as a surgeon working with cancer patients. After completing medical school at the prestigious University of Chicago Pritzker School of Medicine, "Dr. E" completed his general surgical internship, residency, and chief residency at the respected University of California, San Diego, Medical Center. During his resident training, Dr. E spent an additional two years as a Research Fellow in the Surgical Oncology Laboratory, studying cellular membrane function in colon cancer cell lines. A highly sought-after speaker, he has delivered literally hundreds of interactive lectures, both for the medical community and general population during his training at the University of Chicago, the University of California, and the University of Minnesota, and subsequently as a member of the surgical faculty at Stanford University. Dr. E has authored numerous articles and book chapters as well as serving as an editor for a renowned cancer encyclopedia and the senior editor of a book on colon and rectal cancer. He has served in executive roles with venture capital–financed medical device companies and other healthcare businesses. His passion in caring for people diagnosed with cancer expands well beyond the operating room and into the world of the overwhelming emotions, fears, and limited knowledge in which live those with cancer and the family and friends who love them. Visit him at OwnYourCancer.com.